CHAIR YOGA FOR SENIORS

AN ILLUSTRATED GUIDE TO GAIN STRENGTH, IMPROVE MOBILITY, AND LOSE WEIGHT IN 21 DAYS!

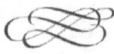

Written by: Rachel Haduch

Chair Yoga Model: Leslie Haduch

Photographer: Richard Haduch

Vitality Solutions Publishing

CONTENTS

RACHEL AND LESLIE HADUCH

Rachel is a dedicated advocate for exercise and healthy living habits. With a passion for promoting wellness at every stage of life, she has spent years cultivating a lifestyle that emphasizes physical activity, balanced nutrition, and mindfulness. As an active woman, Rachel engages in various forms of exercise, including Yoga, Pilates, and strength training, and believes in the transformative power of movement for both body and mind.

Inspired by her mother, Leslie Haduch, a vibrant and active senior, Rachel authored this book on Chair Yoga for Seniors. Her mother serves as the model and muse for the book, showcasing how Chair Yoga can provide a gentle yet effective way for older adults to stay fit, flexible, and independent. Rachel's book is a heartfelt tribute to her mother's vitality and a comprehensive guide designed to help seniors embrace the benefits of yoga, regardless of their mobility levels.

A lifetime artist and active senior, Richard Haduch has been a dedicated photographer for this book, utilizing his eye for detail and light. He has contributed his passion for capturing the beauty of his wife, to help other Seniors also find their beauty within.

As a family this project has been an artistic escapade for all three creators to come together in a shared vision to inspire others to greatness. They are excited to share their collective passion with the world.

BONUS: PRINTABLE EXERCISE CHARTS

Please enjoy these bonus printable exercise charts designed to be used during the 21-Day Challenge. Scan the QR codes to have access to a detailed guide to each week of the Chair Yoga Challenge.

Week 1 Chair Yoga Challenge

Week 2 Chair Yoga Challenge

Week 3 Chair Yoga Challenge

INTRODUCTION: THE SOLUTION FOR SENIORS

Welcome to the Chair Yoga journey of rejuvenation and vitality, specifically tailored for Seniors. In this transformative guide, we invite you to embark on a path to enhance strength, alleviate pain, and foster weight loss—all within the comfort of your home.

Aging is not just about counting the years; it's about embracing life with vigor and resilience. Yet, as we age, our bodies often undergo changes that may challenge our mobility and strength. It's easy to feel disheartened by these physical limitations, but within these pages lies a holistic approach to wellness through rediscovering the joy of movement.

Chair Yoga offers a gentle yet powerful solution, blending the ancient wisdom of Yoga with the accessibility of seated exercises. Regardless of your fitness level or mobility, Chair Yoga empowers you to cultivate flexibility and balance while respecting your body's unique needs and capabilities. By harnessing the breath, performing gentle stretches, and cultivating mindful movement, you'll embark on a journey that transcends physical exercise by nurturing your body, mind, and spirit.

Through targeted sequences and detailed guidance, you'll discover how Chair Yoga can be a powerful tool for sculpting lean muscle, boosting energy levels, alleviating discomfort, and achieving sustainable weight management. This book is more than just a collection of poses and exercises; it's a roadmap for a health transformation. Each chapter has practical tips for integrating Chair Yoga into your day, inspirational stories of Seniors who have excelled in life, and empowering affirmations to support your journey toward optimal wellness. Whether seeking relief from chronic pain, aiming to shed excess pounds, or simply yearning to feel more vibrant and alive, Chair Yoga offers a safe, effective, and enjoyable path to actualizing your health goals.

As you turn the pages and delve into the practices outlined within, remember that you can shape your health destiny. With dedication, patience, and an open heart, you can harness the potential of Chair Yoga to cultivate well-being in your life. So, please take a seat, breathe deeply, and let's embark on this empowering journey together!

THE EVOLUTION OF YOGA INTO CHAIR YOGA FOR SENIORS

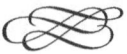

> *"Yoga is not about being flexible; it's about being adaptable."*

— *LAKSHMI VOELKER*

The Goddess Lakshmi is a revered Hindu goddess of abundance and prosperity. Similarly, the Yoga teacher Lakshmi Voelker is a living example of bringing wealth through health to countless Seniors. She has shown us the inspiring influence Yoga can have in the World through her Chair Yoga classes and has trained over 2,500 instructors, creating a widespread movement of adaptive fitness. ("About Lakshmi Voelker", 2022)

Inspired by a student who had a flair-up of arthritis and could not lower herself down to the mat, Lakshmi Voelker developed many of the Chair Yoga poses we use today to enable those who are limited by physical conditions, whether they be from age or injury, to participate in the healing benefits of Yoga. She has been a leader in its development as it has evolved from thousands of years of practice into the form we know today.

YOGA THROUGH THE AGES

In the serene depths of ancient India, amidst the whispers of sages and the rustle of sacred texts, a timeless tradition was born—the practice of Yoga. Rooted in the rich soil of spirituality and philosophy, Yoga emerged as a holistic system for harmonizing body, mind, and spirit. Over millennia, it has evolved and adapted to meet the changing needs of humanity, embracing diverse forms and interpretations. In this chapter, we embark on a voyage through time, tracing the origins of Yoga and its remarkable evolution into Chair Yoga—a gentle yet profound practice tailored for seniors and those recovering from injury.

Origins of Yoga: Unearthing Ancient Wisdom

To understand the essence of Yoga, we must journey back to its origins, deep within the records of Indian history. The word "yoga" derives from the Sanskrit root "yuj," meaning "to yoke" or "to unite." At its core, Yoga is a path of union—the union of individual consciousness with universal consciousness, the union of body with mind, and the union of breath with movement. ("The Yogic Encyclopedia", 2024)

The earliest traces of Yoga can be found in the sacred texts known as the Vedas, dating back over 5,000 years. ("A Brief History of Yoga", 2020) These ancient scriptures, revered as the foundation of Hindu philosophy, contain hymns and rituals to attain spiritual insight and cosmic harmony. Within the Vedas, references to yogic practices such as meditation, mantra recitation, and asceticism abound, laying the groundwork for the development of Yoga as a systematic discipline.

Yoga continued to evolve through the centuries, adapting to India's cultural, social, and spiritual landscape. It flourished within diverse traditions such as Tantra, Hatha Yoga, Bhakti Yoga, Jnana Yoga, and Karma Yoga, each offering unique pathways to self-realization and enlightenment. (McGee, 2022) Yet, amidst this rich tapestry of teachings, the essence of Yoga remained constant—an invitation to awaken to the innate wisdom and potential that reside within each of us.

As centuries passed, the practice of Yoga spread beyond the shores of India, carried by wandering devotees, traveling merchants, and messengers of wisdom. In each new land, it mingled with local traditions, giving rise to hybrid forms of practice and philosophical variation.

The Emergence of Chair Yoga: Meeting the Needs of Seniors

As Yoga gained popularity worldwide, it became increasingly evident that its benefits were not limited to the young and flexible. Many seniors grappling with age-related challenges such as arthritis, osteoporosis, mobility issues, and chronic pain found traditional yoga classes inaccessible or intimidating. Recognizing this unmet need, a new approach to Yoga began to take shape—one that would revolutionize the practice and make it accessible to all.

Chair Yoga emerged as a gentle yet effective alternative, offering modifications and adaptations that catered to the unique needs of seniors and individuals with limited mobility. Rooted in the same principles of breath awareness, mindful movement, and relaxation that underpin traditional Yoga, Chair Yoga creatively reimagined classic poses and sequences to be performed while seated or using the support of a chair.

The pioneering work of yoga teachers such as Lakshmi Voelker-Binder and others paved the way for Chair Yoga's ascent to mainstream recognition. Through innovative techniques and compassionate instruction, they demonstrated that anyone could practice Yoga regardless of age, fitness level, or physical ability. Chair Yoga classes began to increase in community centers, senior centers, retirement homes, hospitals, and yoga studios, offering a sanctuary of healing and empowerment for seniors around the World. ("What is Lakshmi Voelker Chair Yoga?", 2022)

THE ESSENCE OF CHAIR YOGA: MINDFUL MOVEMENT, JOYFUL LIVING

At its core, Chair Yoga embodies the essence of yoga—union, harmony, and self-discovery. It invites seniors to explore the potential of their body and mind, fostering a sense of vitality as well as inner peace. Through the gentle stretches and breath work, Chair Yoga offers a holistic approach to wellness that addresses the physical, emotional, and spiritual dimensions of aging.

In the following chapters, we will delve deeper into the principles and practices of Chair Yoga, exploring its many benefits for seniors and offering practical guidance for integrating Yoga into daily life. From strengthening muscles and improving balance to relieving pain and enhancing emotional well-being, Chair Yoga holds the key to a life of vitality, joy, and fulfillment—at any age.

CREATING YOUR SERENE SANCTUARY

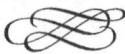

A SAFE SPACE FOR CHAIR YOGA PRACTICE

> *"Peace is always right here. You just have to create space for it."*
>
> — *CAROL TUTTLE*

Tao Porchon Lynch has proven that age doesn't define our abilities. "I believe the key to a long life is positive thinking." She taught. (Lynch, 2021) Before passing at 101 years old, she was entered as the World's oldest yoga teacher in the Guinness Book of World Records. She taught multiple styles of Yoga at the Westchester Institute for Yoga for over 45 years and continued to travel the World teaching yoga workshops well into her 90s. She has inspired us with her dedication to enjoying life, doing Yoga in the mornings, and ballroom dancing in the evenings. She also authored a book about her life's work and her passion to dance through life. Tao Porchon Lynch is proof of her mantra, "There is nothing we can't do if we harness the power within us." ("About Tao," 2017)

THE IMPORTANCE OF SPACE: CULTIVATING TRANQUILITY AND FOCUS

Developing your inner power begins by creating a secure and comfortable environment, where the transformative power of Chair Yoga can blossom. As we embark on this journey of renewal, it is essential to create a sacred space where the body, mind, and spirit can unite in harmony. This chapter will explore creating a tranquil sanctuary for your Chair Yoga practice that nurtures peace, fosters safety, and inspires mindful movement.

Before we unfurl our Yoga mats or settle into our chairs, let us pause to consider the significance of a peaceful space. Our surroundings profoundly impact our state of mind, influencing our ability to relax and connect with the present moment. By cultivating a space free from distractions and filled with a sense of serenity, we create the ideal conditions for deepening our yoga practice.

When selecting a space for your Chair Yoga practice, consider the following factors:

Comfort - Choose a quiet and comfortable area where you feel at ease and can relax fully. Whether it's a spare room, a corner of your living room, or even a tranquil outdoor setting, prioritize comfort and tranquility.

Clutter-Free - Clear away any clutter or unnecessary objects that may distract or inhibit movement. A tidy and uncluttered space promotes a sense of calm and allows for an unhindered energy flow.

Natural Light - Practice in a space that receives ample natural light whenever possible. Natural light uplifts the mood, enhances focus, and fosters a connection with the rhythms of nature.

Ambiance - Set the tone for your practice with soothing elements such as soft lighting, gentle music, or the fragrance of essential oils. Create an ambiance that resonates with your senses and evokes a feeling of relaxation.

Remember that your yoga space reflects your inner sanctuary—a sacred space where you can retreat from the demands of daily life. Take the time to imbue it with intention, creating a haven of healing and renewal.

SAFETY FIRST: ENSURING A SECURE AND SUPPORTIVE ENVIRONMENT

Safety is paramount in any yoga practice, especially for seniors and individuals with limited mobility. By taking proactive measures to create a secure and supportive environment, we can minimize the risk of injury and promote a sense of confidence and empowerment in our practice. Here are some guidelines for ensuring safety during your Chair Yoga sessions:

Stable Seating - Choose a sturdy chair with a flat seat and backrest, preferably without arms. Ensure the chair is positioned on a stable surface, such as a non-slip mat or carpet, to prevent it from sliding or tipping during practice. In many of the exercises we will recommend the chair be pushed against a wall to ensure the chair is a stable platform.

Clear Pathways - Keep pathways clear of obstacles and tripping hazards to facilitate safe movement in and out of yoga poses. Remove loose rugs, electrical cords, and other potential dangers from the practice area.

Adapted Props - Utilize props such as yoga mats, yoga blocks, bolsters, and blankets to provide support and enhance comfort during practice. Props can help seniors modify poses to suit their individual needs and abilities, reducing strain and promoting proper alignment.

Mindful Movement - Move mindfully and at your own pace, respecting your body's limit and avoiding forceful or abrupt movements. Listen to your body and honor any sensations of discomfort or pain.

Modifications and Variations - Utilize the various modifications and variations offered with many poses to tailor the practice to your unique needs and abilities. If you have any questions or concerns, consult your doctor.

By prioritizing safety as our highest goal, you can feel empowered to engage in Chair Yoga with confidence and ease, enabling you to reap the full benefits of your practice while minimizing the risk of injury or strain.

GROW AT YOUR OWN PACE: MODIFICATIONS FOR ANY NEED

We have created these workouts as a guide to attaining your best self, but this goal looks different for each person, and we encourage you to personalize your Chair Yoga workout to fit your individual needs. Utilize the modifications if you are meeting any strain or pain in the body and formulate your workout plan to allow you to grow without compromising your body's abilities.

We face change in our bodies as we age, often surfacing in our spine, shoulders, hips, and knees as a lifetime of productivity can take a toll. You may be navigating the challenges of arthritis, osteopenia, osteoporosis or recovering from knee or hip surgery. Exercises that focus on these sensitive parts of the body can help but they can also aggravate the joints and muscles. As every situation is different, begin slow and gradually work your way up to build your resilience and strength.

When a pose feels challenging, slowly explore the sensations that it creates. The first time you try the pose it may not look like the picture, but your body is adaptable, often becoming more flexible even after the first few times you try it. Do not become discouraged after trying a pose for the first time, instead try again the next day and see how creating a reoccurring workout routine can greatly benefit your body in the long term.

Many exercises featured will offer a modification. If you suffer from low blood pressure, avoid exercises that place your heart above your head to prevent dizziness. If you have joint pain, exercise slowly to prevent pain or potential accidents, especially those requiring bending repetitions in sensitive areas. Preexisting conditions such as Osteopenia or Osteoporosis benefit from exercise through improved bone mass and reduced risk of falling. Take your time when approaching an exercise that has a modification to avoid injury.

If you wish to take your workout to the next level, increase the repetitions. The fitness level of the exercises is geared towards the most accessible number of repetitions but if the posture and position of the exercise inspire you and feel especially beneficial for your body, repeat the exercise and breathe deeper into the pose!

In your Yoga space, you can discover a refuge of peace and presence—a sacred oasis where you can nourish your body, mind, and spirit in harmony. Let us create a sanctuary of healing and renewal where we can retreat from the noise and busyness of the World and reconnect with the wisdom and beauty that dwell within.

THE POWER OF BREATH

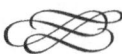

CENTER YOUR MIND TO DEEPEN YOUR PRACTICE

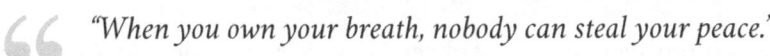

"When you own your breath, nobody can steal your peace."

— *ANONYMOUS*

Vivian Stancil has inspired those who didn't believe they could improve their health. Through her remarkable journey, she exemplifies the transformative power of physical activity. At the age of 19, Vivian developed a degenerative ailment in her eyes, causing her to lose her eyesight. When she turned 50, her doctor told her that she would not live past her 60th birthday because she was significantly overweight and had developed a heart murmur. ("My Story", 2024)

The sound of water had always soothed her, so she decided to explore swimming because other forms of physical activity seemed too challenging with her blindness. Even though she was scared to let go of the wall when entering the pool, she pushed past her fear, losing over 100 pounds and eliminating her heart murmur. Now, she competes in many races, including the Special Olympics. Her infectious laugh and inspiring story have motivated many people to prioritize their well-being and follow an active lifestyle. "If something is too hard, I'm still going to work at it until I get it." We can overcome all obstacles if we focus on bettering our bodies. (Levy, 2021)

THE PEACE WITHIN OUR CONSCIOUS BREATH

In the gentle rhythm of our breath lies a profound gateway to presence and peace. As we embark on our Chair Yoga journey, let us explore the importance of mindful breathing—an invitation to awaken to the wonder of each moment. We will highlight the principles of conscious breathing and discover how it can enhance our Chair Yoga practice, fostering vitality and relaxation.

Yoga is often seen as a very physical exercise practice, focusing on the "asanas" or postures, and the benefits that they bring to the body. People usually overlook the powerful practice of slowing the breath and finding peace in the stillness.

At its core, mindful breathing brings focused awareness to the breath, anchoring ourselves in the present moment with each inhalation and exhalation. Conscious breathing has been a simple yet profound path to inner peace for thousands of years. By cultivating this mindfulness, we can observe our thoughts, emotions, and bodily sensations with clarity and compassion, releasing ourselves from the grip of past regrets and future anxieties.

Take a few moments to scan through your body, bringing gentle awareness to each area from head to toe. Notice any areas of tension or discomfort and invite them to soften and release with each exhale. Approach this practice with curiosity and acceptance, allowing thoughts and sensations to arise without attachment or aversion. Embrace whatever comes up for you with compassion, knowing each moment is an opportunity for growth and self-discovery.

By harnessing the power of the breath, seniors can enhance their vitality, reduce stress, and cultivate a sense of calm in their daily lives. Moreover, mindful breathing can be adapted to suit individual needs and abilities, making it accessible to practitioners of all ages and fitness levels. We can find the strength to be our best selves in these peaceful moments.

EXPLORING THE BREATH: DIFFERENT FORMS OF PRANAYAMA

Within the vast landscape of Yogic practices, there exists a technique for refining mindful breathing known as pranayama—literally, "control of the life force." (Everheart, 2024) These ancient practices offer a spectrum of tools for harnessing the breath and channeling its energy for healing, relaxation, and spiritual awakening. Pranayama also serves as a potent vehicle for fostering a deeper connection with the inner self.

Let's explore some of the primary forms of pranayama that can enrich your Chair Yoga practice:

DIAPHRAGMATIC BREATHING (DIRGHA PRANAYAMA)

Also known as "three-part breathing," this technique involves consciously engaging the diaphragm to expand the belly on inhalation and contract it on exhalation. Diaphragmatic breathing promotes relaxation, reduces stress, and enhances blood oxygenation, making it an ideal practice for seniors seeking to cultivate a sense of calm and well-being. ("Three-Part Breath", 2023)

1. Begin with a good posture, seated with your spine aligned. Relax your shoulders, keeping them down and away from your ears. Place your feet hip-width apart for stability. Close your eyes to increase focus on the breath.

2. Place one hand on your heart and one hand on your stomach. Take a slow, deep breath in through your nose. As you inhale, feel your abdomen expand and rise. Imagine filling a balloon in your belly.

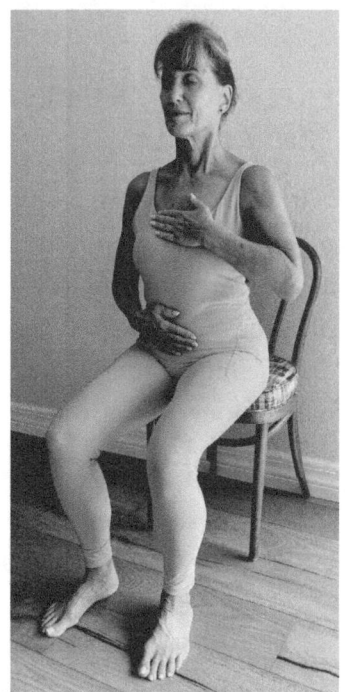

Diaphragmatic Breath Step 2

3. Exhale slowly and evenly through your mouth, allowing the air to flow naturally. Feel your abdomen gently contract and lower as you exhale all the air out of your lungs without straining.

4. On the next inhale, once the abdomen fills, continue inhaling to fill the thoracic area under the rib cage. Exhale all air out of the abdomen and rib cage.

5. As you breathe in again, consciously engage your diaphragm, rib cage, and upper chest. Feel it expand with your breath. Exhale the breath out in reverse order, releasing the upper chest, the rib cage, and the abdomen.
6. Ensure that you remain relaxed throughout the practice. Tension in your neck, shoulders, or jaw may indicate shallow breathing.
7. Continue this diaphragmatic breathing pattern for 10 repetitions. Gradually extend the duration as you become more comfortable.

ALTERNATE NOSTRIL BREATHING (NADI SHODHANA)

This balancing pranayama technique involves alternating between the left and right nostrils while breathing, gently using the fingers to close one nostril at a time. Alternate Nostril breathing helps harmonize the body's energy flow, clears the mind, and promotes mental clarity and focus. It is particularly beneficial for seniors experiencing anxiety, insomnia, or imbalances in the nervous system. (Cronkleton, 2023)

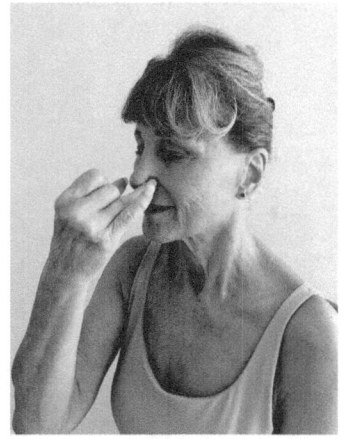

1. Sit in a comfortable position with your spine straight, and your shoulders relaxed.
2. During this exercise, use your right thumb to close your right nostril and your right ring finger to close your left nostril. Fold your pointer and middle fingers down towards your palm.

Alternate Nostril Breathing Step 4

3. Closing your right nostril, Inhale through your left nostril for a count of four.
4. Close your left nostril and release your right nostril.
5. Exhale through your right nostril for a count of four.
6. Inhale through your right nostril.
7. Close your right nostril and release your left nostril.
8. Exhale through your left nostril.
9. Continue for 10 repetitions of this breath, alternating between nostrils.

UJJAYI BREATHING

Commonly referred to as "ocean breath" or "victorious breath," Ujjayi breathing involves constricting the back of the throat slightly to create a soft, whispering sound during inhalation and exhalation. This rhythmic breathing technique calms the mind, regulates the nervous system, and enhances concentration, making it an excellent practice seeking mindfulness and inner peace. (EkhartYoga, 2024)

1. Begin seated tall with your hands resting on your thighs.
2. Inhale deeply in through the nose, constricting the back of the throat to make the sound of the waves crashing on the shore.
3. Exhale steadily out through the nose with the same continuous sound.
4. Breathe evenly, creating a rhythmic loop without breath retention.
5. Continue for 10 ocean breaths.

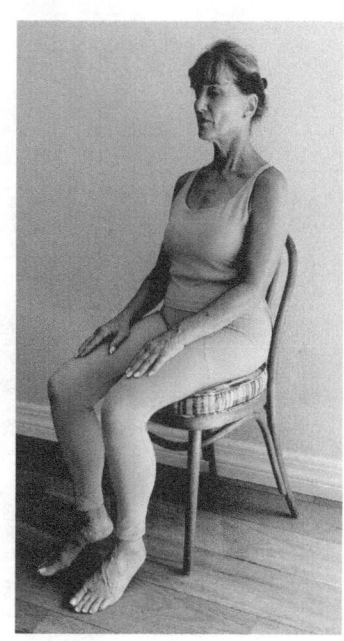

Ujjayi Breath Step 2

SITALI BREATHING

In this cooling pranayama technique, practitioners curl the tongue into a "straw" shape, inhaling deeply through the mouth and exhaling through the nostrils. Sitali breathing has a soothing effect on the body and mind, calming emotions and promoting relaxation. It is especially beneficial for people experiencing hot flashes, anxiety, or digestive issues. (Ekhart, 2023)

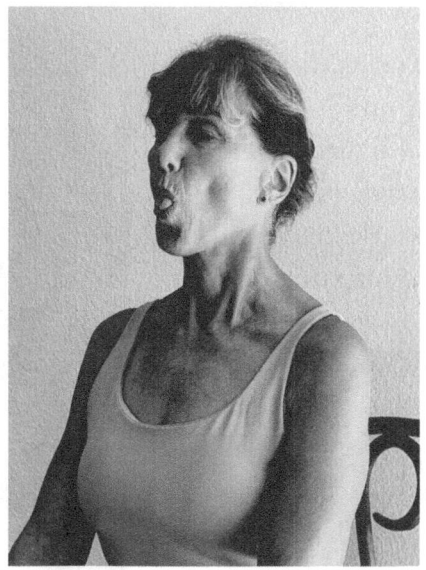

Sitali Breathing Step 2

1. Begin seated with a good posture and relaxed shoulders.
2. Curl the tongue by bringing the sides of the tongue up into a taco shape.
3. Inhale for the count of 4.
4. Hold your breath for the count of 2.
5. Close your mouth and exhale all your breath through the nose for a count of 4.
6. Continue for 10 repetitions.

BHRAMARI BREATHING (BEE BREATH)

This calming pranayama technique, named after the buzzing sound of a bee, soothes the nervous system by promoting a sense of inner peace. It is a great practice to quiet the mind and cultivate deep relaxation. (Husseiny, 2022)

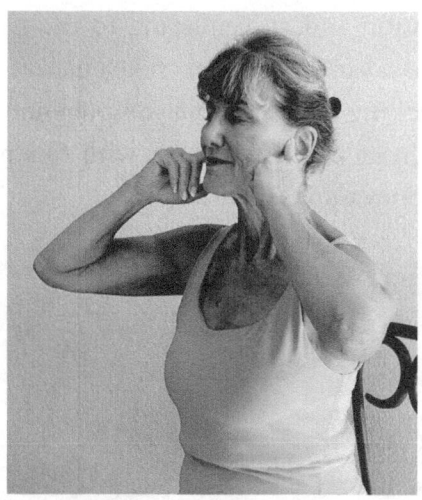

Bee Breath Step 2

1. Close your eyes and plug your ears with your fingers to keep out external sound.
2. On the inhale, take a deep breath through the nose.
3. Exhale slowly while creating a gentle hum, like the buzzing of a bee, in the back of the throat throughout the full exhale.
4. Continue for 10 repetitions of Bee Breath.

SHAVASANA (CORPSE POSE)

While not a breathing technique, Shavasana is a profoundly restorative posture that allows practitioners to integrate the benefits of breathing (pranayama) and postures (asanas). You can even practice Shavasana in your chair if you cannot lie on the floor. While reclining comfortably with eyes closed, focus on sinking into deep relaxation and surrendering to the natural rhythm of your breath. Shavasana promotes rejuvenation and integration into the body, making it an essential component of any Chair Yoga practice. Often, Yoga classes will end with this pose in the cool-down. ("Corpse Shavasana", 2023)

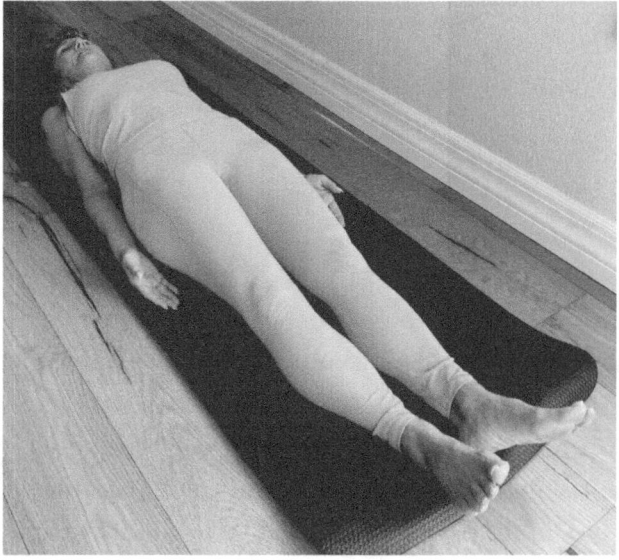

Shavasana Step 3

1. Lay in a relaxed position on your mat or sit in a chair if it's more comfortable. It should be a place to feel fully supported while relaxing all your muscles. Use a blanket to ensure you are warm and comfortable, so you don't get a chill after building up heat during your practice.

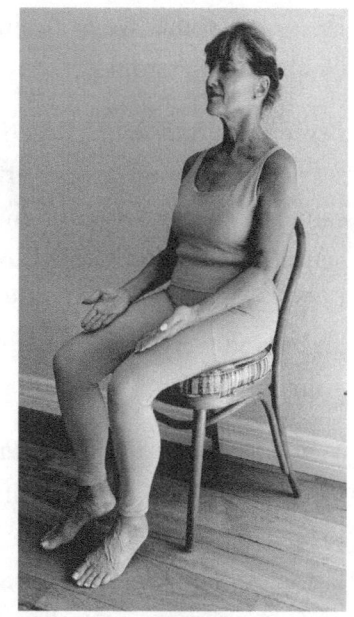

Shavasana Modification

2. Allow your arms to fall open from your body with your palms facing up at a 45-degree angle.

3. Close your eyes and take long, deep breaths through the nose. Letting your body become heavy and releasing tension as you sink into the floor as you exhale.

4. Stay in this position for 2 minutes or until you feel completely relaxed and rejuvenated.

Experiment with these different techniques to discover which resonates most deeply with your body, mind, and spirit, and remember to approach your practice with patience, curiosity, and an open heart.

Here are some ways to integrate mindful breathing into your Chair Yoga sessions:

Begin and End with Breath Awareness - Start each Chair Yoga session by bringing your attention to the breath, anchoring yourself in the present moment with mindful awareness. Notice the sensations of the breath flowing in and out of the body without judgment or effort. At the end of the session, savor the stillness and tranquility that arises from deepening your connection with your breath.

Sync Movement with Breath - Coordinate movement with breath to create a seamless flow of energy and awareness throughout the practice. Synchronize each movement with an inhalation or exhalation, moving mindfully and with intention. By linking breath and movement, we cultivate presence and focus, enhancing the mind-body connection and promoting a sense of ease and fluidity in our practice.

Use the Breath as an Anchor - During challenging poses or moments of discomfort, use the breath as an anchor, guiding you back to the present moment with each inhalation and exhalation. The breath is a constant source of support and guidance, providing a refuge of peace and stability amidst the fluctuations of the mind and body.

Practice Breath Awareness Throughout the Day - Cultivate mindfulness of the breath beyond the confines of your Chair Yoga practice, integrating it into your daily life. Take moments throughout the day to pause and bring your attention to the breath, whether waiting in line, sitting in traffic, or enjoying a quiet moment at home. We cultivate a more profound sense of presence and resilience by weaving breath awareness into the fabric of daily life.

CHAIR YOGA WARM-UP

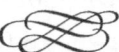

ENERGIZE YOUR BODY, AWAKEN YOUR SPIRIT

"You are only one workout away from a good mood."

— *CAROLINE JORDAN*

Johanna Quass qualified as the oldest competitive gymnast in the World in 2012. At age 86, she specialized in the parallel bars, the beam, and the floor routines, doing handstands and flips with a smile! Even though she no longer competes due to an injury in 2018, she continues to stay active, impressing many with her ability to stand on her head and play soccer at 96. (Sienra, 2023)

This passion for gymnastics began at the young age of 10, and she has pursued this passion throughout her life as a coach and a competitor. For many years, she focused her athletic abilities on handball competition, and at 57, she again began to compete in gymnastics. She says, "My face is old, but my heart is young." It is a testament to an active lifestyle's energizing and enriching qualities. (Natale, 2020)

GENTLE BEGINNINGS IN MOVEMENT

Just as the morning sun gently awakens the earth, a well-designed warm-up sequence prepares your body and mind for the transformative journey of your workout and into your day. For seniors, a gentle and mindful warm-up is essential to ensure safety, comfort, and optimal performance throughout the practice. It bridges stillness and movement, inviting you to tune into your breath and reconnect with your body. Whether you're a seasoned yogi or new to this practice, the warm-up offers a gentle start to your practice to honor your body's needs.

Proper posture and balance ensure safety and alignment throughout our practice. A balanced posture supports optimal functioning of the body's systems, promotes efficient movement, and fosters a sense of confidence and well-being. Alternately, poor posture can lead to many health issues, including back pain, joint stiffness, muscle tension, and reduced mobility. ("Why Good Posture Matters", 2017)

Balance is not merely a physical attribute; it is a dynamic interplay of strength, flexibility, and proprioception—the body's awareness of its position in space. Maintaining balance becomes increasingly important as we age to prevent falls, maintain independence, and promote overall well-being. Fortunately, our Chair Yoga warm-up offers a variety of practices to help seniors cultivate stability in their bodies.

The warm-up loosens tight muscles and improves joint mobility, making moving into and holding yoga poses easier with proper alignment. It helps release tension and stiffness, allowing you to experience greater freedom of movement and flexibility in your practice.

By gently mobilizing your joints, warming up your muscles, and increasing blood flow to your tissues, the warm-up helps reduce the risk of injury during your practice. It prepares your body for the physical demands of Yoga, ensuring that you can move with ease throughout the session.

Center yourself in the present moment, and let the warm-up guide you as you step onto the path of Chair Yoga with mindful movement.

SEATED MOUNTAIN POSE (TADASANA)

Align the spine into proper posture and center the mind for the beginning of your Chair Yoga practice.

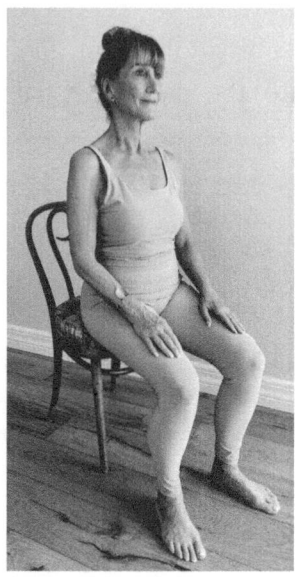

Seated Mountain Step 1

1. Begin by sitting tall in your chair with your feet flat on the floor and your spine straight. Place your hands on top of your thighs.
2. Ground down through your sit bones and lengthen through the crown of your head. Stack one vertebra on top of the other to feel your spine elongate.
3. Draw your shoulders back and down, opening your chest and allowing your breath to flow freely through the nose and mouth. You can close your eyes for a deeper calm.
4. Hold the pose for 5 breaths, feeling a sense of alignment in your spine.

PRAYER POSE

Center your balance and find peace in your heart.

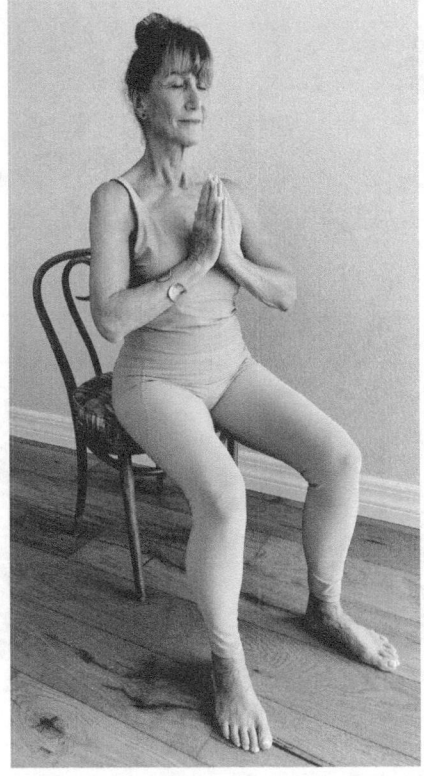

Prayer Pose Step 3

1. Begin seated with feet flat on the floor and a tall posture.
2. Bring your palms together before your heart, relaxing your shoulders down your back.
3. Take 5 deep breaths in this position, closing your eyes to center your breathing and create presence in your body.

NECK ROTATIONS

Feel a gentle stretch in the neck and shoulders.

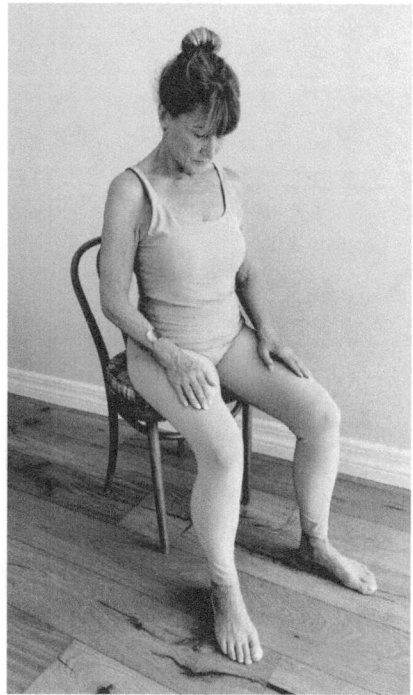
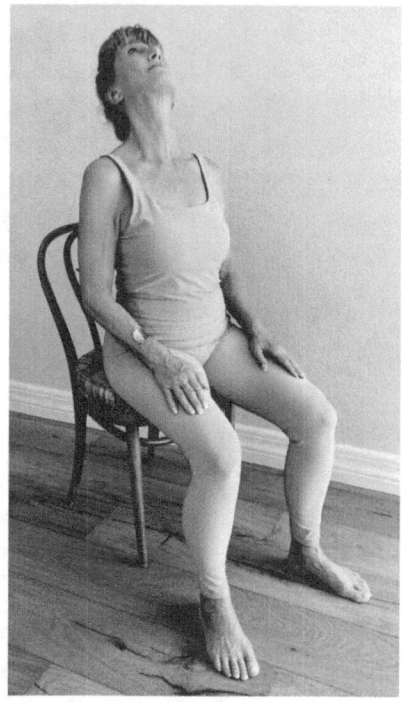

Neck Rotation Step 2   *Neck Rotation Step 4*

1. Begin seated with your palms resting on your thighs.
2. Tilt the head towards the chest and take a deep breath.
3. Rotate the head, bringing the left ear to the left shoulder. Take a deep breath.
4. Tilt the head back so you are looking up at the ceiling. Take a deep breath.
5. Rotate the head, bringing the right ear to the right shoulder. Take a deep breath.
6. Repeat this full rotation 2 more times.

SHOULDER ROTATIONS

Find release in the shoulders and relax the muscles in the back.

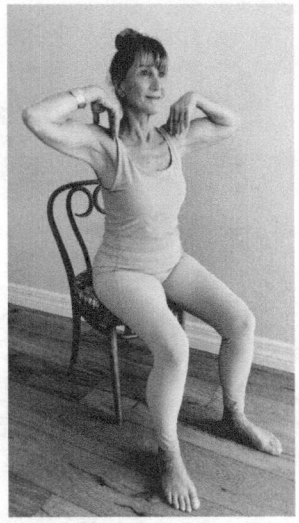

Shoulder Rotations Step 2

1. Begin seated on the edge of your chair for full Range of Motion in your upper body with your feet flat on the ground.
2. Place your left fingertips on your left shoulder and your right fingertips on your right shoulder.
3. Rotate your elbows in a circular motion, bringing the elbows forward, then down and back, then up and forward. **Modification**: Rotate one shoulder at a time to create a gentler stretch.
4. Breathe in through the nose and out through the mouth as you continue this exercise 5-10 times.
5. Rotate the elbows in a circular motion in the opposite direction, bringing the elbows back, down, and forward, then up, back, and down for 5-10 rotations.

CAT-COW POSE

Stretch your spine and back muscles for flexibility and balance in posture.

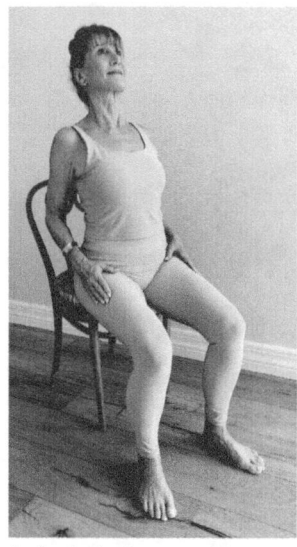 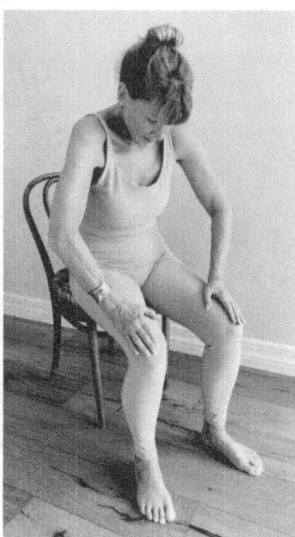

Cat Cow Pose Step 2   Cat Cow Pose Step 3

1. Sit tall in your chair with your feet flat on the floor and your hands resting on your thighs.
2. Inhale, arching your back and lifting your chest, allowing your ribs to move forward and your head to tilt back.
3. As you exhale, round your spine and tuck your chin towards your chest, drawing your navel towards your spine. Place your fingertips on your knees as you round your back.
4. Flow smoothly between these two positions, syncing your breath with your movement.
5. Continue for a total of 10 repetitions.

MARCHING EXERCISE

Mobility in the hips and strength in the core and legs.

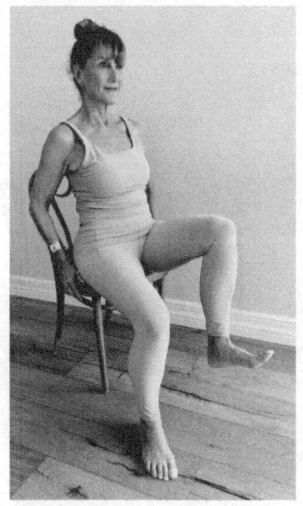

Marching Step 2

1. Begin seated at the edge of your chair, holding onto the chair seat to stabilize yourself through the exercise.
2. Inhale and raise your left knee, flexing your foot to engage the leg. Exhale and lower to the ground in a controlled motion. **Modification** – If you have had hip or knee surgery, lift the foot only as far as you are comfortable.
3. Inhale and raise your right knee, flexing your foot to engage the leg—Exhale and lower to the ground in a controlled motion.
4. Breathe deeply through the nose and out through the mouth as you continue the exercise for a total of 10 repetitions. Keep a good rhythm of marching to match your breathing.

TOE HEEL RAISES

Lengthen the muscles in the calf and ankles while finding balance throughout the body.

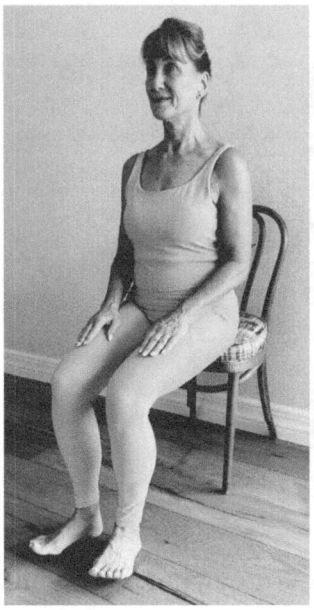 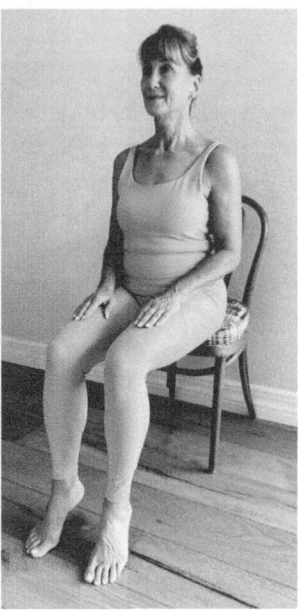

Toe Heel Raises Step 2   *Toe Heel Raises Step 4*

1. Begin seated on the edge of your chair with your hands resting on your thighs and your spine elongated.
2. Inhale as you lift your toes.
3. Exhale as you lower your toes.
4. Inhale as you lift your heels, rising onto the balls of your feet.
5. Exhale as you lower your heels.
6. Continue for 10 repetitions of the exercise.

ARMS REACH

Open the upper body and shoulders; find a balanced posture.

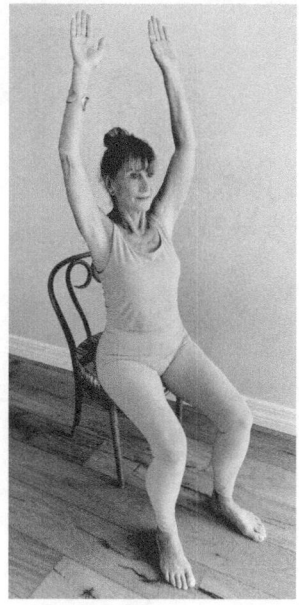

Arm Reach Step 2

1. Begin with your feet flat, sitting with the back straight and tall and your palms on your knees.
2. On the inhale, lift the arms up and over the head.
3. Exhale and keep your arms raised, relaxing the shoulders.
4. Take another deep breath in through the nose, reaching your fingertips up to the ceiling.
5. Lower your hands to your knees as you exhale through the mouth.
6. Continue for 5 total repetitions of this stretch.

SIDE BEND

Create flexibility in the shoulders and length in the spine.

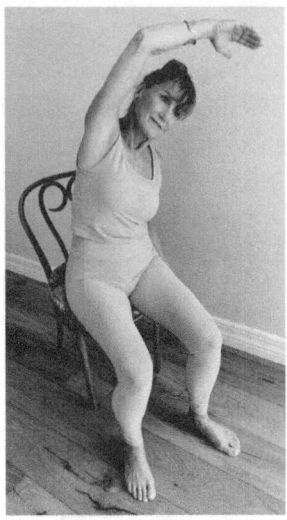

Side Bend Step 2

1. Begin seated with your left hand holding the left side of the chair.
   Modification- Place your hand on your thigh for a lighter shoulder stretch.
2. Inhale and lift the right arm, extending the arm over the head to the left for 3 breaths, inhaling through the nose, and exhaling out of the mouth.
3. Bring your right arm down to hold the side of your chair with your right hand.
4. Inhale and lift the left arm, extending the arm over the head to the right for 3 breaths, inhaling through the nose, and exhaling out of the mouth.
5. Bring your left arm down to grip the left side of the chair.
6. Continue for 2 more repetitions on each side.

SIDE TWIST

Stretch the spine and lengthen through the torso, creating aware-ness of proper posture.

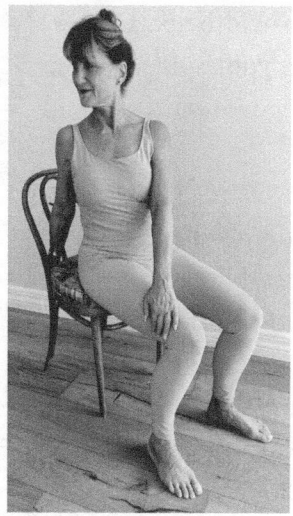

Side Twist Step 3

1. Sit tall in your chair with your feet flat on the floor and your spine elongated.
2. Place your right hand on the back of the chair seat and your left hand on your right knee. **Modification**- For a gentler stretch in the spine, hold the side of your chair and turn only as much as is comfortable for your body.
3. Inhale to lengthen your spine, then exhale to twist gently to the right, using your hands for support.
4. Hold the twist for 3 breaths, inhaling through the nose while stretching the spine and exhaling out of the mouth while deepening the twist.
5. Repeat on the other side, placing your left hand on the back of the chair seat and twisting to the left.
6. Continue this twist for 2 more repetitions on each side.

FORWARD FOLD

Find length in the spine and a gentle stretch in the hips.

1. Sit tall at the edge of your chair with your feet hip-width apart.
2. Inhale to lengthen your spine, then exhale to hinge forward at the hips.
3. Bring your chest towards your thighs and your forehead towards your knees, allowing your hands to hold your legs as you lower down. Your hands may land on your calves or even lower to the ground. **Modification**: Fold forward as far as your hips and spine will allow. If you suffer from low blood pressure, keep your head above your knees so you don't get dizzy. Brace yourself by clasping your hands together and resting your forearms on your thighs.
4. Hold the pose for 3 even breaths, feeling a gentle stretch along the back of your body.
5. When returning to the seated position, slowly raise yourself, stacking your vertebrae one at a time.

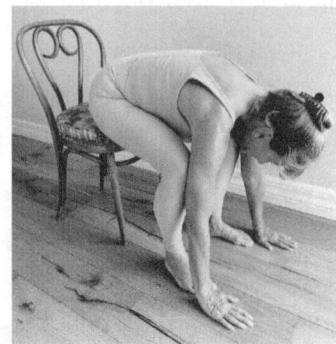

Forward Fold Step 3

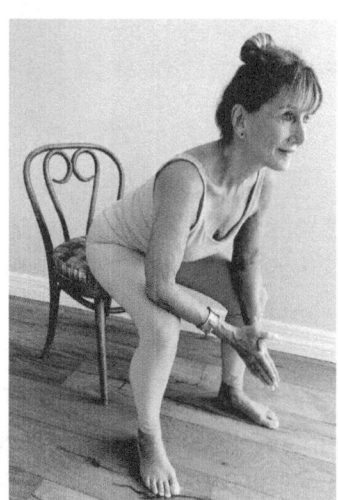

Forward Fold Modification

BEGINNER POSTURES

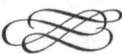

BUILDING A STRONG AND STABLE FOUNDATION

 "Nothing will work unless you do."

— *MAYA ANGELOU*

I t doesn't take professional training to begin a journey of reaching your goals. Joann Sampson is a Senior Games speed runner who drives forward with resilience. After she retired from being an elementary school teacher, she began competitively running at the age of 62 without any previous athletic experience. After reading about the Senior Games in her local newspaper, Joann registered for her first race, winning a gold medal in her very first race! She began running five days a week and doing Yoga in the evenings to build her stamina. (Sampson, 2022)

At 83, she won 3 gold medals at the Delray Beach Senior Games in sprinting, and countless medals in the 20 years she has been competitively running. She reaches this level of success through hard work and commitment to her practice. Now, as a motivational speaker, she says, "All you have to do is believe in yourself since you are the only one who can stop you." ("Hallandale Beach Resident Leads the Way," 2022)

LAYING THE GROUNDWORK WITH BEGINNER EXERCISES

To meet your personal goals, you must start at the beginning. These foundational Chair Yoga postures serve as the building blocks of your practice, providing stability and support for more advanced poses. Beginner poses aid in developing strength and flexibility, empowering you to move confidently during and after your workout.

Practicing beginner postures allows you to cultivate awareness of proper alignment and body mechanics. You can refine your practice by paying attention to your body's posture cues and sensations. These foundational postures incorporate elements of balance and coordination, challenging you to find flexibility in your movement and gently stretching your muscles.

Practicing these poses with care can reduce the risk of falls and injury, enhancing your confidence in everyday activities. We will explore a selection of foundational Chair Yoga postures for the whole body, also offering modifications to accommodate a range of abilities and needs. These postures will help you establish a strong and stable foundation for your practice, empowering you to explore the transformative benefits of Yoga with confidence and ease.

CHEST OPENER

Stretch the arms and shoulders, open the ribs, and find length in the spine.

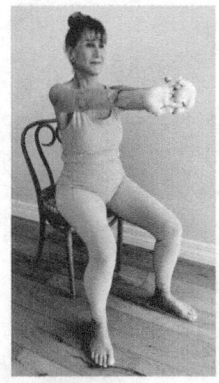 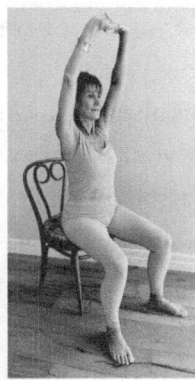

Chest Opener Step 2   *Chest Opener Step 4*

1. Sit with a straight back in your chair with your feet flat on the ground.
2. Lift your arms straight before you with your fingers interlaced and your palms facing away.
   Modification- If it is uncomfortable to interlace your fingers, have one hand hold the other hand.
3. Inhale as you push your hands away from you, dropping your shoulders down your back.
4. Exhale as you pivot your arms up and over your head, keeping your arms straight and opening the chest to create a slight arch in your back.
5. Inhale and slowly bring your arms down to shoulder height.
6. Continue for 5 total repetitions.

CRESCENT MOON POSE

Flexibility through the ribs while stretching the shoulders.

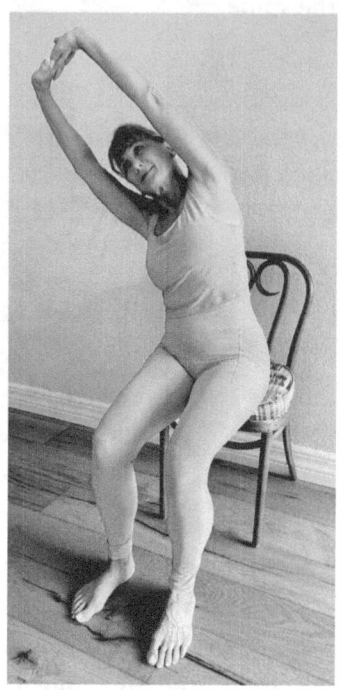

1. Start seated with your spine elongated and your feet flat on the floor before you.
2. Lift your arms above your head and interlock your fingers with your palms facing the ceiling.
3. Inhale and extend the spine, lengthening and stretching your arms to the sky.
4. Exhale and bend at the ribs, stretching to the right side, moving only your upper body and keeping your arms straight.
5. Hold for 3 deep breaths, Breathing in through the nose and out through the mouth.

Crescent Moon Step 4

   Modification – Hold this pose for as many breaths as is comfortable. Start with one breath and work your way up to 3 even breaths.
6. Inhale and stretch back up to the center with your arms reaching high.
7. Exhale and bend at the ribs, stretching to the left side with straight arms.
8. Hold for 3 deep breaths, breathing in through the nose and out through the mouth.
9. Inhale and stretch back up to the center.
10. Repeat this exercise once more on each side.
11. Exhale and release your arms down slowly.

SPHINX POSE

Strengthening the spine, improving the posture, and opening the chest.

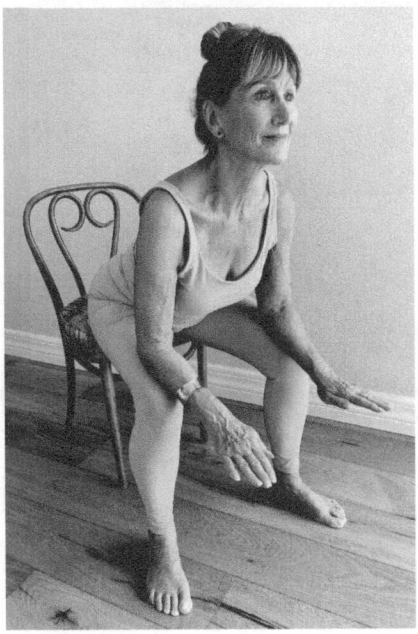

Sphinx Pose Step 3

1. Sit with an aligned posture and your feet flat on the floor in front of you.
2. Bring your forearms down to your thighs, resting your weight on your knees.
3. Arms are facing forward with palms facing down.
4. Arch your back, bringing your navel to your thighs and opening your chest so your head lifts.
5. Hold this pose for 10 deep breaths. Inhaling through the nose and exhaling through the mouth.

SPINAL TWIST WITH ARM REACH

Create flexibility in the spine and mobility in the shoulders.

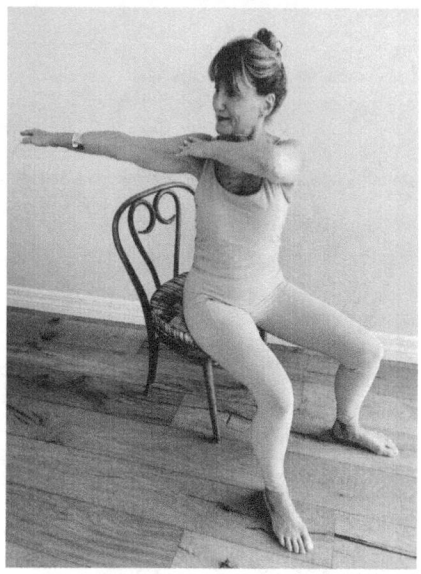

Spinal Twist with Arm Reach Step 2

1. Sit with your spine elongated and your feet grounded on the floor.
2. Turn to your right, placing your left hand on your right shoulder.
3. Extend your right arm straight out as far as possible to the right at shoulder height.
4. Inhale and lengthen the spine.
5. Exhale and gently push your shoulder with your left hand, deepening your stretch.
6. Continue for 5 breaths, then return to the center.
7. Repeat the stretch on the left side of the body.

BACK STRETCH

Strengthening the mid back and stretching the chest.

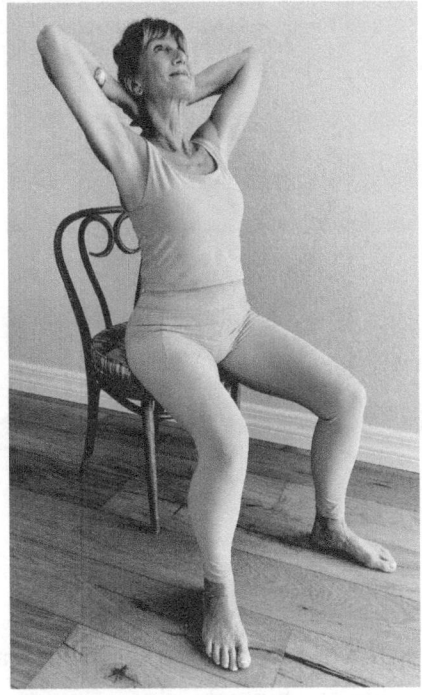

Back Stretch Step 3

1. Sit on the edge of your chair with your feet flat on the ground before you. Feet shoulder width apart.
2. Lift your arms to interlock your fingers behind your neck with your elbows extended to either side of your head.
3. Take 3 deep breaths as you tilt your head back to look at the ceiling.
4. Bring your head forward to look at your navel to stretch the back in the opposite direction.
5. Repeat this exercise 2 more times.

HIP CIRCLES

Create flexibility in the hips while loosening tension in the spine.

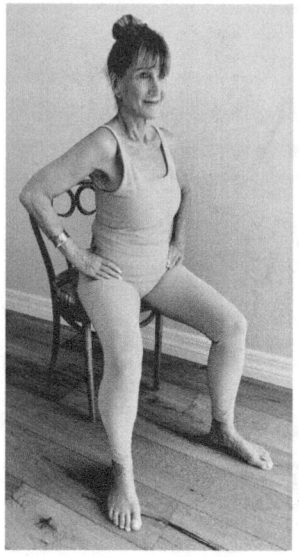

Hip Circles Step 2

1. Start seated with your feet flat on the ground and your hands resting on your hips.
2. Rotate the hips to the right in a clockwise circle, exaggerating the movements to deepen the stretch.
3. Keep the upper body still as you isolate the movement of the core and hips.
4. Continue to breathe evenly, Inhaling through the nose and out through the mouth.
5. Continue for 5 total repetitions with a clockwise movement.
6. Switch directions for 5 repetitions of a counterclockwise movement.

SUPPORTED SQUATS

Open the hips and create mobility in the legs.

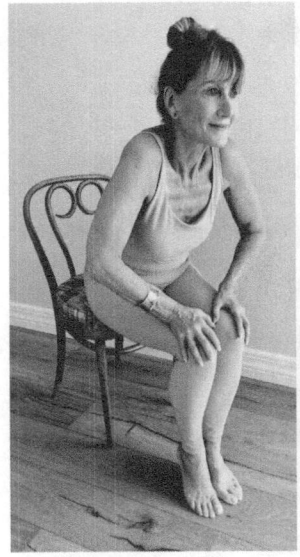 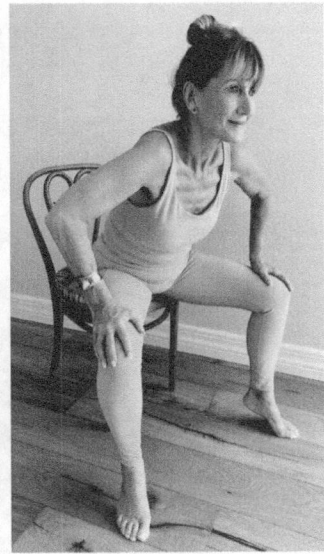

Supported Squats Step 1   *Supported Squats Step 2*

1. Sit on the edge of your seat, balanced on the balls of your feet and your hands resting on your knees.
2. On your inhale, open your knees so that they are at a 90-degree angle from each other.
3. On the exhale, rock your body to balance as you gently jump your feet together to bring the knees back to the center.

   Modification - For those with sensitive hips or knees, or those with osteoporosis; instead of opening both knees simultaneously, rotate one knee at a time, keeping the breath even.
4. Continue for 5 repetitions.

SIDE LEG RAISES

Improve balance and posture while improving leg strength.

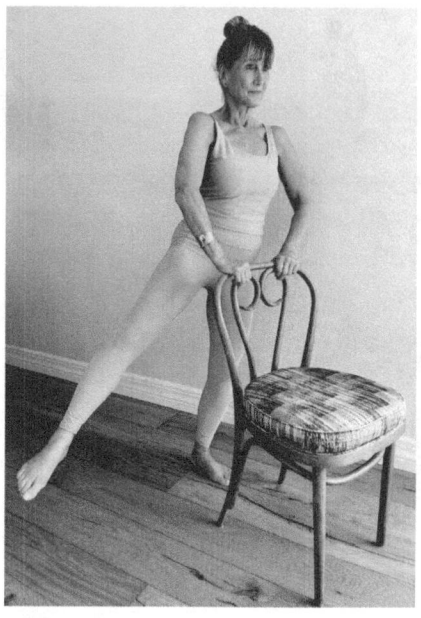

Side Leg Raises Step 2

1. Start by standing behind the back of your chair with both hands supporting you.
2. On the Inhale, lift the right foot to the right side about 12 inches off the ground.
3. On the exhale, lower the foot with controlled movements, bringing it back to your side but not touching the ground.
4. Continue with this motion a total of 5 repetitions.
5. Repeat this exercise with the left leg raising and lowering.

WARRIOR I POSE

Builds stamina as you elongate the torso and strengthen the hips.

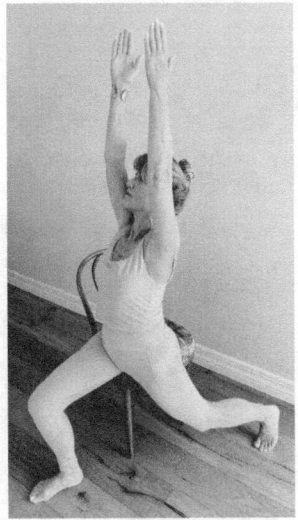

Warrior I Pose Step 3

1. Sit tall at the edge of your chair with your feet hip-width apart.
2. Inhale to lift your arms overhead, reaching up towards the sky with your palms facing each other.
3. Exhale to bend your left knee towards the ground and pivot to face your torso to the right.
4. Keep your right foot planted on the floor and your spine elongated while your left foot faces forward.
5. Hold the pose for 5 breaths, then return to neutral.
6. Repeat this posture facing the left.

STANDING KNEE TAPS

Strengthen the core and legs while benefiting balance and coordination.

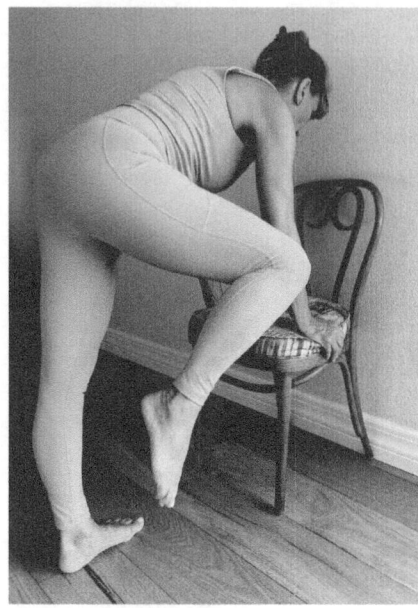

Standing Knee Taps Step 3

1. Stand facing the seat of your chair with <u>the back of the chair up against the wall to stabilize the pose</u>.
2. Bend down to grip each side of the chair seat.
   Modification– If you have challenges bending over, complete this exercise while standing behind the chair and lifting your knees as comfortably as possible.
3. Inhale as you lift your right knee towards your right elbow, getting as close as possible to tapping your knee.
4. Exhale and lower your foot back down to the ground.
5. Continue for a total of 5 repetitions on the right leg.
6. Switch sides to knee tap on the left side for 5 repetitions.

CHAIR LUNGE

Gain balance while opening the hips and stretching the hamstrings.

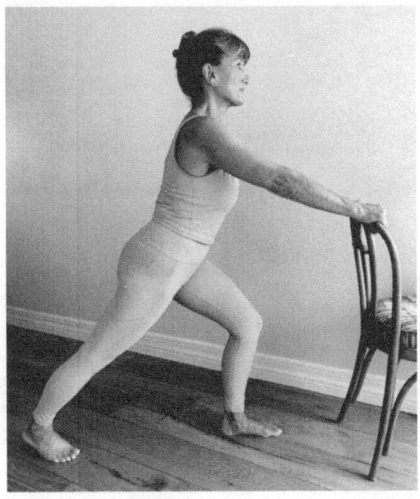

Chair Lunge Step 3

1. Stand behind the back of your chair while holding on with both hands. Push the seat of the chair against the wall to stabilize the stretch.
2. As you inhale, relax your shoulders.
3. Exhale and step back 2 feet with your right foot so that it is facing forward.
4. Bend your left knee, keeping your knee directly above your ankle with your hips facing forward.
5. Hold this pose for 5 breaths. Inhale through the nose, exhale through the mouth.
6. Step back to standing.
7. Switch sides to step back with the left leg.

INTERMEDIATE POSES

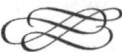

DEEPENING YOUR PRACTICE, EXPANDING YOUR HORIZONS

> *"The reason I exercise is for the quality of life I enjoy."*
>
> — *KENNETH H. COOPER*

L ife often presents us with challenges and bodily injuries as we age, particularly for those leading active lifestyles. But does this mean we surrender our physical aspirations and dreams? Not for Kathy Meares. Despite enduring four knee surgeries, she persists in competing and pushing her limits. Sports have been a significant part of her life, with 4-5 mile runs as a morning ritual. When a doctor advised her to put less stress on her knees, Kathy faced disappointment. Yet, she chose resilience over resignation: "I can either sit here and whine about how I can't do it, or I'm gonna get out there and get started and work my way up to what I need to be doing." Determined, she gradually rebuilt her strength through daily walks. Discovering a power walking event at the National Senior Games sparked her inspiration and Kathy triumphed, winning first place in her inaugural competition. Since then, she has not only claimed numerous victories but has also captured hearts with her unwavering commitment to staying active. (Levy, 2021)

ENHANCE YOUR PRACTICE BY EXPLORING YOUR ABILITIES

As you progress along your Chair Yoga journey, you may feel more comfortable and confident in your practice. You may notice a deeper connection to your body and breath or less joint pain. Intermediate poses offer an opportunity to challenge yourself, step out of your comfort zone, and continue to grow and evolve on your yoga journey.

Chair Yoga is an opportunity to refine your alignment and deepen your breath awareness as you delve deeper into the transformative benefits of Yoga. Whether you're seeking to build strength, enhance flexibility, or enrich your practice, these poses provide a pathway to greater well-being with modifications to accommodate a wide range of abilities and needs.

Remember to approach these poses with openness and self-compassion as you explore them. Listen to your body's wisdom and honor its unique needs and limitations. If a pose feels uncomfortable or inaccessible, don't hesitate to modify or skip it altogether. Enjoy the time you are granting yourself for self-care as you engage your body in this beneficial practice.

PIGEON POSE

Create a deep stretch in the hips and flexibility in the legs.

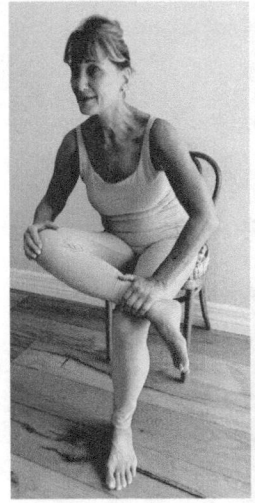 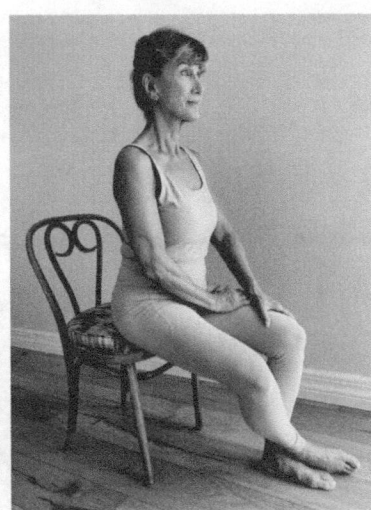

Pigeon Pose Step 2   *Pigeon Pose Modification*

1. Sit tall in your chair with your feet flat on the floor.
2. Cross your right ankle over your left knee, flexing your right foot. Place both hands on your knee to gently stretch further.
3. Inhale to lengthen your spine, then exhale to hinge at the hips, bringing your chest towards your right shin.
   Modification – For a gentle stretch for the hips, cross the right ankle over the left ankle.
4. Keep your back flat and your shoulders relaxed.
5. Hold the pose for several breaths, feeling a deep stretch in your right hip.
6. Return to the center and repeat Pigeon Pose on the other side.

COBRA POSE

Open the chest and elongate the spine.

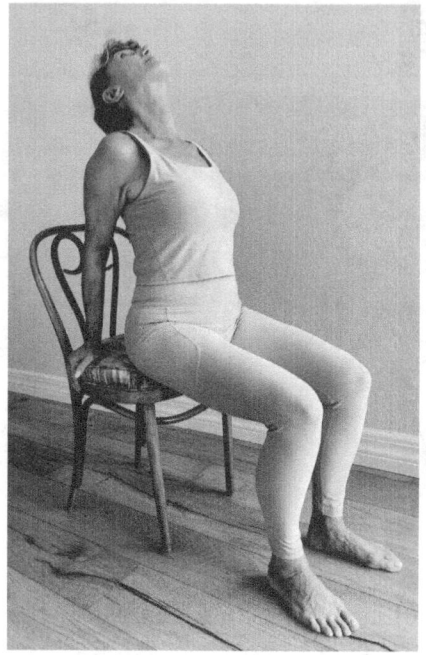

Cobra Pose Step 3

1. Begin by sitting tall at the front of the chair.
2. Place your hands behind you on the seat of the chair.
3. Inhale and tilt your head back, lifting your chest while keeping your neck relaxed.
4. Hold the position for 5 breaths, breathing in through the nose and out through the mouth.

EAGLE ARMS

Stretch the upper back and shoulders.

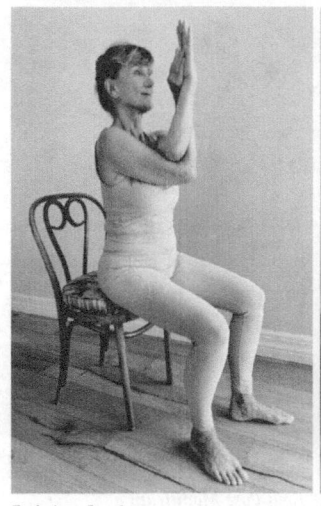 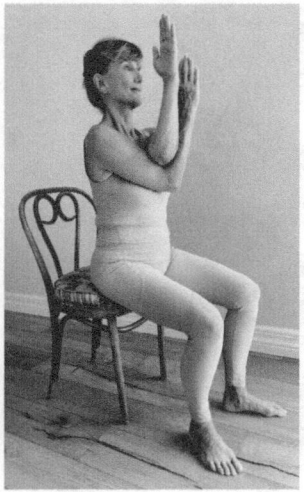

Eagle Arms Step 3   *Eagle Arms Modification*

1. Sit tall in your chair with your feet flat on the floor.
2. Inhale to reach your arms out to the sides, then exhale to cross your right under your left arm, wrapping your forearms and bringing your palms together.
3. Exhale and lift your elbows, relaxing your shoulders away from your ears.
   Modification- If there is shoulder pain when wrapping the arms, cross the arms and lift without bringing palms together.
4. Hold the pose for 5 breaths, inhaling through the nose and out through the mouth.
5. Repeat on the other side, crossing your left arm under your right arm and holding for 5 breaths.

BOAT POSE

Stability in the core and strength in the legs.

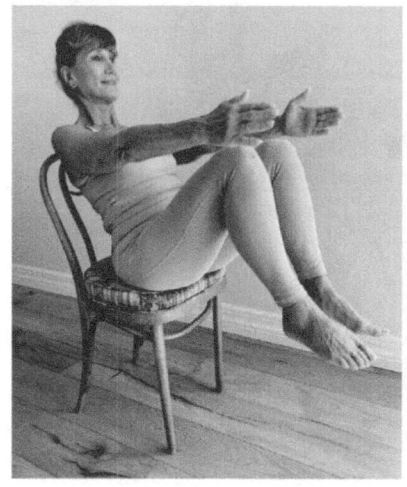 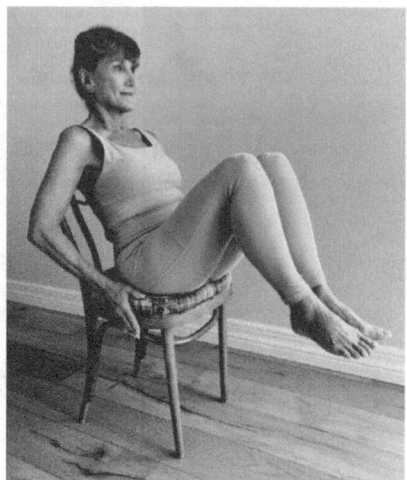

Boat Pose Step 4   *Boat Pose Modification*

1. Sit tall at the edge of your chair with your feet flat on the
   floor and your hands resting on your thighs.
2. Inhale to lengthen your spine.
3. Exhale to lift your feet off the floor, lean back on the chair
   to balance on your sit bones, bringing your knees (as far as
   is comfortable for you) towards your chest to engage the
   core.
   Modification: To aid in balance, hold onto the edges of the
   chair as you bring your knees up towards your chest.
4. If you are confident in your sense of balance, you can
   extend your arms alongside your legs.
5. Hold the pose for 5 breaths, feeling a sense of strength and
   stability in your core.

CHAIR SQUATS

Ground down through the legs and create stability in the core.

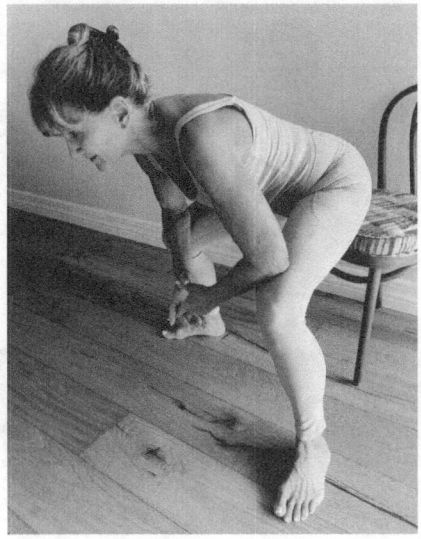

Chair Squats Step 2

1. Begin at the edge of your chair with your feet flat on the floor and your feet in a widened stance.
2. Lean forward to brace your forearms on your knees with your hands interlocking. On the inhale, lean forward, balancing your weight between your feet as you balance in the squat position.
3. Continue even breathing as you hold the pose for the count of 5.
4. Lean back into the chair to rest.
5. Continue the squats for 3 total repetitions.

PLANK POSE

Increase stability within the whole body, strengthening the core.

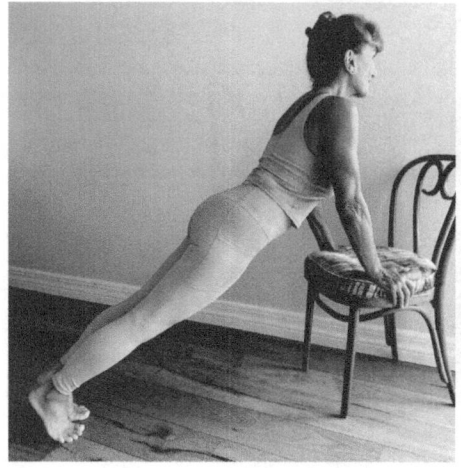 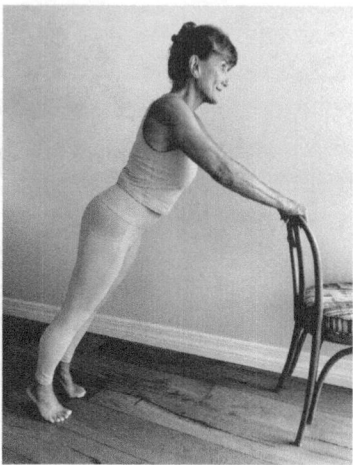

Plank Pose Step 3   *Plank Pose Modification*

1. Begin by standing in front of your chair. <u>Brace the chair against a wall so the chair does not slide</u>.
   Modification- If you need a more accessible stretch on your shoulders, perform this posture standing behind the back of your chair.
2. Lean down so both hands are on the edge of your chair seat.
3. Step back from the chair so you are on the balls of your feet, forming a straight line from your neck down your spine to your feet. Engage your core.
4. Hold this position for 10 even breaths.

MOUNTAIN CLIMBERS POSE

Building muscle in the core and back, bringing mobility to the hips and legs.

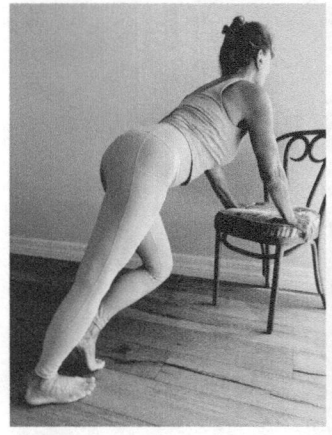 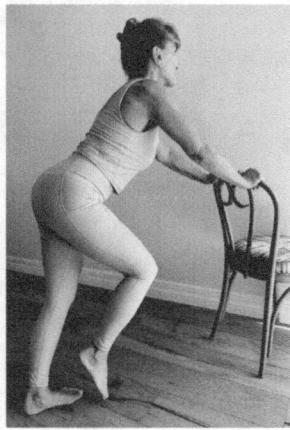

Mountain Climbers Step 4   *Modification*

1. Begin standing facing the seat of the chair. <u>Brace the chair against the wall to ensure a stable surface</u>.
   Modification- For a more accessible stretch on the arms and shoulders, perform this posture standing behind the chair, holding onto the backrest.
2. Lean down so both hands balance on the edge of your chair.
3. Step back from the chair so that you are on the balls of your feet, forming a straight line from your neck, down your spine, to your feet.
4. Lift the heels of your feet as you jog in place, bringing your knees forward slightly as you keep your breathing even.
5. Keep the core muscles engaged throughout the motion.
6. Continue this motion for 10 total breaths.

DANCER'S POSE

Open the shoulders and stretch through the hip and spine

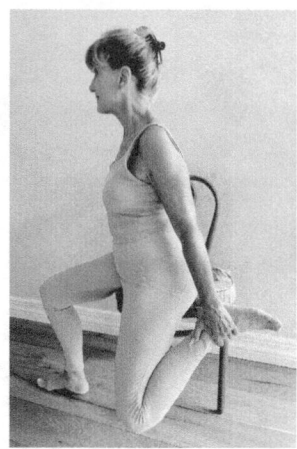

Dancers Pose Step 3

1. Begin seated at the edge of your chair.
2. Rotate your body to the right and bring your right foot to the right side of your chair. Hold onto the back of your chair with your right hand.
3. Reach down with your left hand and grab above your ankle, dropping your left knee towards the floor. Stretch tall in your spine, dropping your shoulders down your back.
   Modification- Use a pillow underneath your left knee to support your leg and place less stress on your hips and knees. Also optional is a strap that you can loop around your ankle and hold with your left hand.
4. Hold this pose for 5 breaths.
5. Repeat this pose with your right leg.

TRICEPS DIPS

Strengthen the arms while toning the core.

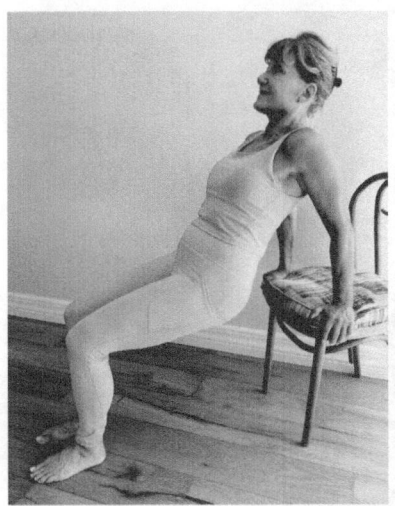 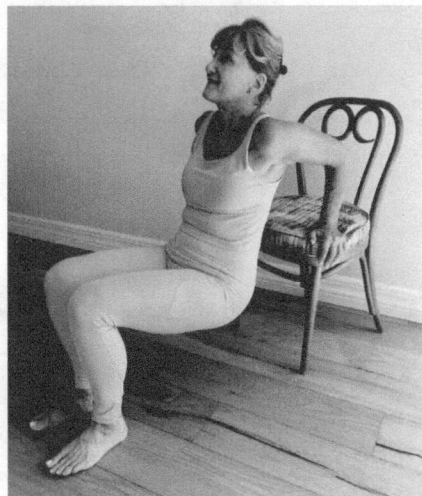

Triceps Dips Step 2   *Triceps Dips Step 3*

1. Begin seated on the edge of your seat with a tall posture and your chair braced against the wall.
2. Grip the sides of the chair as you step your feet forward six inches, ensuring they are stable.
3. Inhale, lifting your hips forward off the seat and bending at the elbows, bringing your hips down towards the ground.
4. Exhale and straighten your arms to bring your hips up.
5. Continue for 5 repetitions.

TRIANGLE POSE

Increase mobility in the hips and lower spine, stretching the muscles in the thigh.

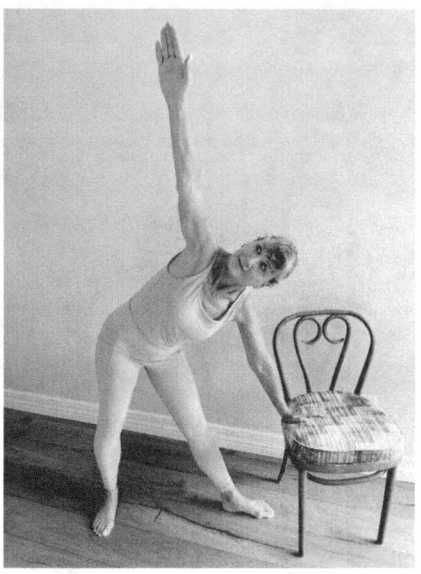

Triangle Pose Step 5

1. Begin standing with the seat of the chair on your left side.
2. Widen the stance of your feet so they are about 2 feet apart, your right foot facing forward and your left foot facing the chair.
3. Bend to your left side so your fingertips touch the seat of your chair, keeping your legs straight.
4. Raise your right arm straight above your head.
5. Turn your head to gaze up at your fingertips.
6. Take 5 breaths in this pose.
7. Move to the right side of the chair to repeat on the other side of the body.

LEG LIFTS

Strength in the core and increased balance throughout the body.

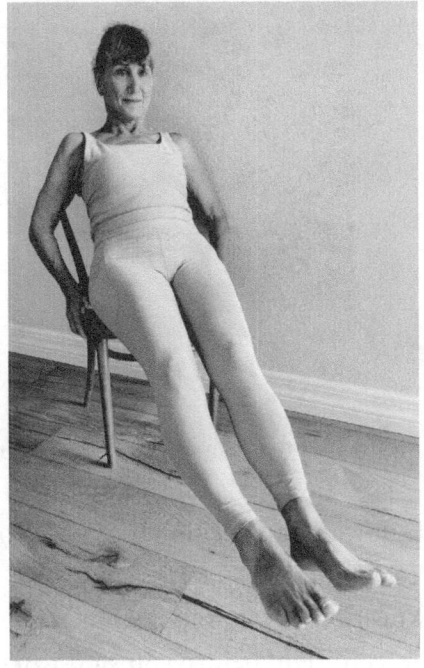

Leg Lifts Step 2

1. Begin seated in your chair with your legs extended out before you.
2. Hold the sides of your chair as you lean back to raise your legs off the ground about 2-6 inches.
3. Hold for a count of 5, slowly lowering your legs on the exhale.
4. Repeat 2 more times. Try to hold the pose longer with each repetition.

CHAIR POSE

Enhance balance and improve hip and knee mobility.

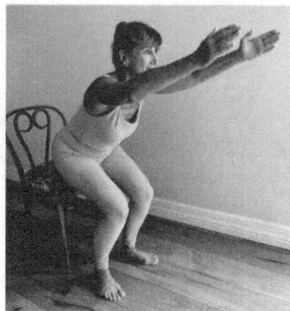

Chair Pose Step 3

1. Begin standing in front of the chair as if you are going to sit down.
2. As you inhale, lower yourself slowly, with your arms stretched before you.
3. Bend at the knee, keeping both knees facing forwards.
4. Pause your descent right before you sit down in the seat of the chair.
5. Hold the pose for the count of three, continuing to breathe evenly throughout the pose.
   Modification- This pose may be too challenging on the knees to hold the pose, so it is optional to lower down to the seat, practicing the raising and lowering motion from seated.
6. On the inhale, raise to standing, pushing your feet into the ground to raise to standing.
7. Continue for 4 more repetitions. Hold the pose longer with each hold if possible.

DOWNWARD DOG

Create length in the spine and stretch the whole body, from the shoulders to the calves.

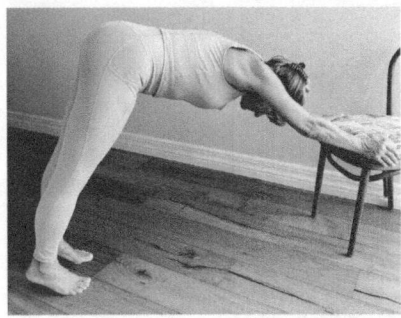
Downward Dog Step 3

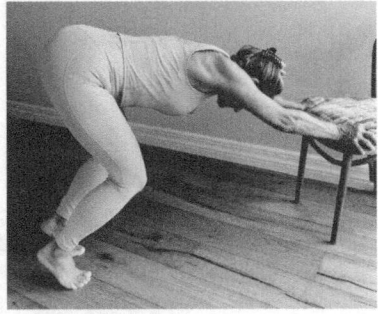
Downward Dog Modification

1. Stand facing the seat of your chair. Ensure the chair is stable and will not slip by placing the back of the chair against the wall.
2. Bend down to grasp the edges of the chair seat with both hands.
3. Keep your arms by your ears, creating a straight line from the arms to the hips, hinging at the hips so that the body forms a "V" shape.
   Modification- To put less pressure on the knees, create more of a bend in the knee.
4. Allow the knees to relax so there is a slight bend; sink the heels into the ground to feel a stretch in your hamstrings.
5. Hold for a count of 5.

UPWARD PLANK

Create strength in the arms and shoulders while improving mobility in the hips.

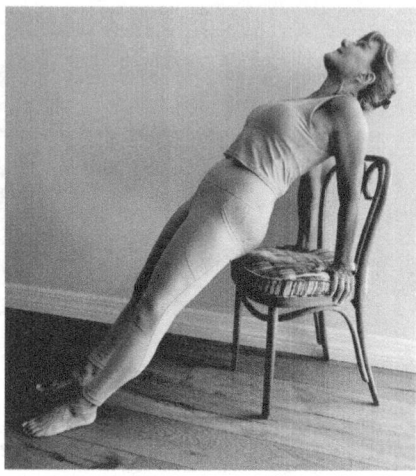

Upward Plank Step 3

1. Start seated on the edge of your chair, placing your hands behind you on the seat while gripping the sides.
2. Extend your legs in front of you with your feet flat on the ground.
3. On the inhale, transfer your weight into your hands and feet as you lift your hips off the chair, creating a straight line from your feet up to your head.
4. Maintain even breathing in through the nose and out through the mouth as you hold the pose to the count of 5.
5. Keep your neck and jaw relaxed as you slowly lower back to the chair.
6. Repeat this pose 2 more times.

BUTTERFLY POSE

Create strength in the core while challenging the balance of the body.

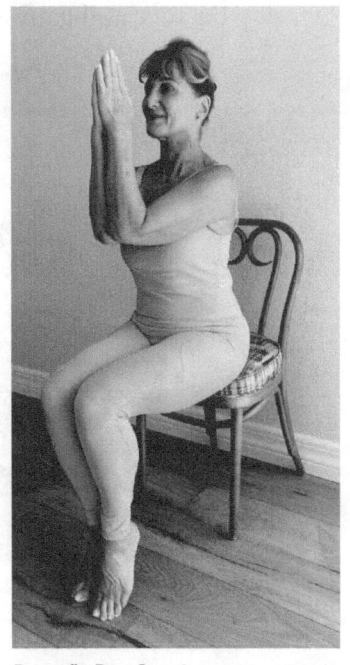

Butterfly Pose Step 2

1. Begin seated at the edge of your chair with your balance on the balls of your feet.
2. Bring the arms up before the face with elbows bent at a 90-degree angle.
3. Take a deep inhale through the nose.
4. As you exhale, lean back to open the arms and legs to either side of the body, keeping your elbows raised and your feet off the ground.
5. Inhale, bringing the arms and legs back together, balancing on the balls of your feet.
6. Open and close the arms and legs in unison with the breath for 3 repetitions. Return to the center on your toes.
7. Repeat 2 more times.

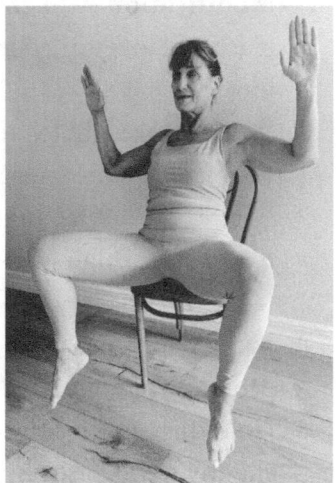

Butterfly Pose Step 4

WARRIOR II POSE

Develop balance and gain strength in the legs.

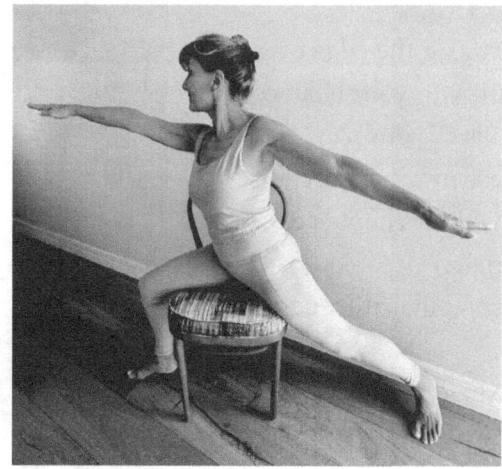

Warrior II Step 4

1. Begin seated on the edge of your chair.
   Modification – To create a gentler stretch in the hips, place a blanket or rolled-up mat on the chair to elevate the hips.
2. Swing your right leg to the right side of your chair so that your calf is at a 90-degree angle.
3. Extend the left leg to the left side of the chair so that the top of your thigh is on the chair's seat and your toes are facing forward.
4. Bring your arms up to create a T so they are parallel to the ground, your gaze looking past your right hand.
5. Hold this pose for the count of 5-10. You may lift your hips slightly to hover over your chair to intensify the stretch.
6. Repeat this pose on the other side of the body.

ADVANCED POSES

ELEVATING YOUR PRACTICE, EMBRACING TRANSFORMATION

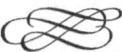 *"Don't stop until you're proud."*

— *VINCE LOMBARDI JR.*

P at Lillihei discovered a new purpose when she left her career as a stockbroker, reinvesting her time and energy into her health and well-being. At 71, she insists, "There is fun after 70. I'm having more fun than I've ever had, and I'm healthier than I've ever been." Encouraged by her daughter in 2008, she entered a 150-mile bike race. Despite finishing last, her sense of achievement was profound. Undeterred, she pursued a triathlon next, focusing on training and strength-building, resulting in weight loss and more energy. Since embracing an active lifestyle, she has shed 50 lbs. and conquered over 18 triathlons. Her belief that "motion is medicine" is a testament that transformative change is achievable at any age. (Blount, 2015)

TAKING YOUR PRACTICE TO THE NEXT LEVEL

When your body feels comfortable with the essential Chair Yoga poses, you can explore advanced poses to challenge your body and expand your practice to new heights. While the journey of Yoga is never-ending, advanced poses offer an opportunity for seniors to explore their physical and mental capabilities, fostering resilience and empowerment.

As you continue your Chair Yoga practice, you may find yourself drawn to challenging poses that test your strength, flexibility, and balance. Advanced poses invite you to push beyond your comfort zone, confront your limitations, and discover the untapped potential within you. These poses build upon the foundation established by beginner and intermediate postures, offering a deeper exploration of self-awareness.

Advanced poses require greater strength, flexibility, concentration, and willingness to embrace discomfort and uncertainty. They invite you to confront your fears, break through barriers, and tap into your inner reservoir of resilience and courage. While some poses may seem daunting initially, they offer an opportunity for transformation when approached slowly and with respect for your body.

Remember to approach advanced poses with curiosity and self-compassion. If a pose feels too challenging or inaccessible, modify or skip it altogether. The goal is not to achieve perfection but to engage wholeheartedly with the present moment and the experience it brings.

UPWARD DOG

Elongate the spine and strengthen the shoulders.

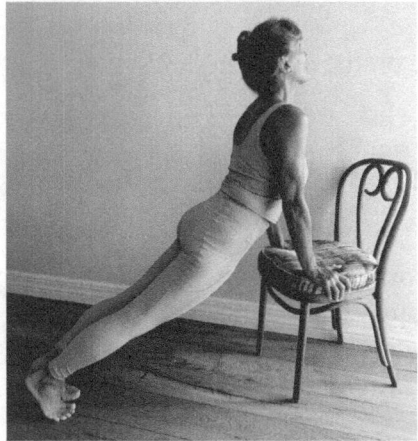

Upward Dog Step 4

1. Begin standing in front of the seat of your chair. <u>Ideally, the back of the chair should be pushed against the wall to eliminate slipping</u>.
   Modification- Use the back of the chair for this exercise to give a gentler stretch in the spine.
2. Bend down and grip either side of the chair seat.
3. Step back into plank pose so your spine is straight from your head to your feet.
4. Lower your hips towards the chair's seat and raise your gaze to look forward. Keep your arms straight, and your shoulders relaxed down.
5. Hold this pose for the count of 5, continuing breathing evenly throughout the exercise.
6. Slowly step back to the chair. Repeat this pose 2 more times.

EXTENDED SIDE ANGLE

Create length in the spine while toning the core and strengthening the legs.

1. Begin seated on the edge of your chair.
2. Rotate your right leg to the right side of your chair, facing your foot to the right. Straighten your left leg to the left of your chair and face your left foot forward. Align the heel of your right foot to the arch of your left foot.

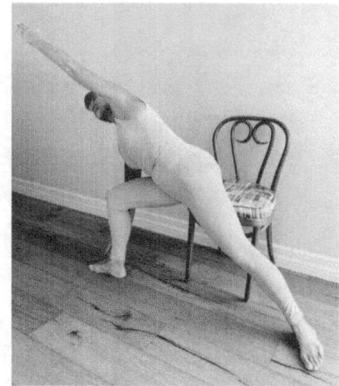

Extended Side Angle Step 3

3. Reach your right hand to your right foot and stretch your left arm over your head to point right. Breathe slowly and evenly through the stretch. **Modification**- For a gentler stretch in the spine and hips, rest your right elbow on your right knee and stretch your left arm over your head to the right side.
4. Hold for the count of 5.

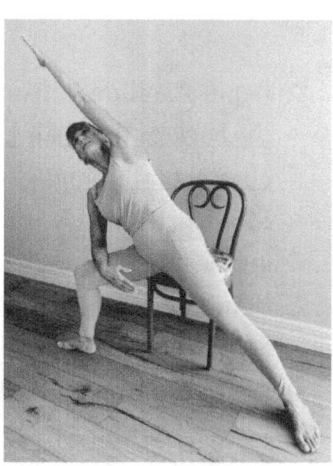

Extended Side Angle Modification

5. Reposition your body to stretch the other side. The left foot should face the left, and the right foot should face forward to stretch the right side of the body.

GATE POSE

Open the hips and stretch the legs while finding length in the spine.

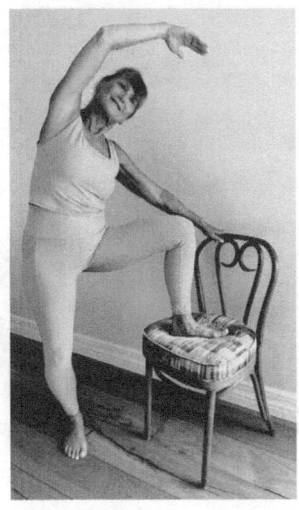

Gate Pose Step 3

1. Stand so that your left side is in front of the seat of your chair.
2. Lift your left foot onto the chair seat, stabilizing yourself to ensure you don't fall by facing your right foot forward.
3. Place your left hand on the back of your chair and inhale, reaching your right arm up and over your head.
4. Hold the pose for 10 breaths, breathing steadily as you stretch towards the left.
5. Repeat this posture with your right foot on the chair, stretching to the right.

LOW LUNGE

Create a deep stretch in the hips and knees while practicing balance.

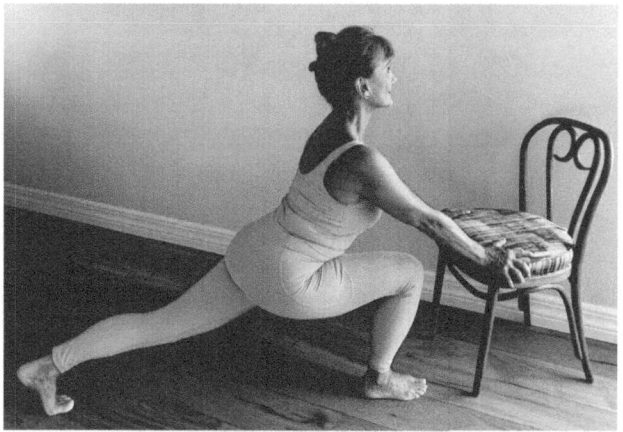

Low Lunge Step 2

1. Begin standing, facing the front of your chair, with your feet shoulder distance apart.
2. Hold onto the seat of your chair as you step back with your left foot, lowering your hips slowly as you bend your right knee, keeping your knee over your ankle. Keep your chest lifted and your front foot flat on the ground.
3. Face your left foot forward as you balance for 10 breaths. **Modification** – Instead of dropping so low, keep a slight bend in the knee for a lighter stretch in the hips.
4. To safely exit the pose, lean forward, put your weight onto your hands, and push up with your legs.
5. Repeat the low lunge on the other side of the body with the left knee bending and the right leg stepping back.

THREE-LEGGED DOWNWARD DOG

Stretch the hips and challenge the balance.

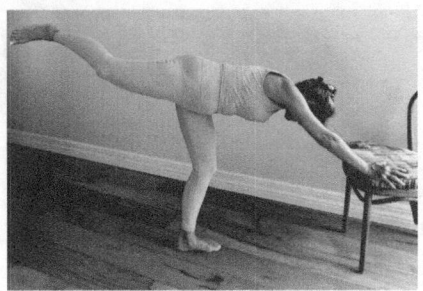

Three-Legged Downward Dog Step 4

1. Begin standing in front of the seat of your chair. <u>Push the back of the chair against the wall to brace the chair</u>.
2. Bend and place your hands on the edges of your chair to stabilize yourself.
   Modification – Place your forearms on the seat of the chair to make balancing easier.
3. Lower your head between your arms, keeping them straight as you lift your hips.
4. Lift the right leg off the ground behind you and raise it as high as you feel comfortable.
5. Hold to the count of 3, breathing in through the mouth and out through the nose.
6. Slowly lower your leg back to the ground.
7. Lift the left leg off the ground as high as you feel comfortable and continue to breathe evenly.
8. Hold to the count of 3 and slowly lower to the ground.
9. Repeat the 3-Legged Downward Dog 2 more times on each leg.

WARRIOR III POSE

Cultivate balance and leg strength as you stretch the spine.

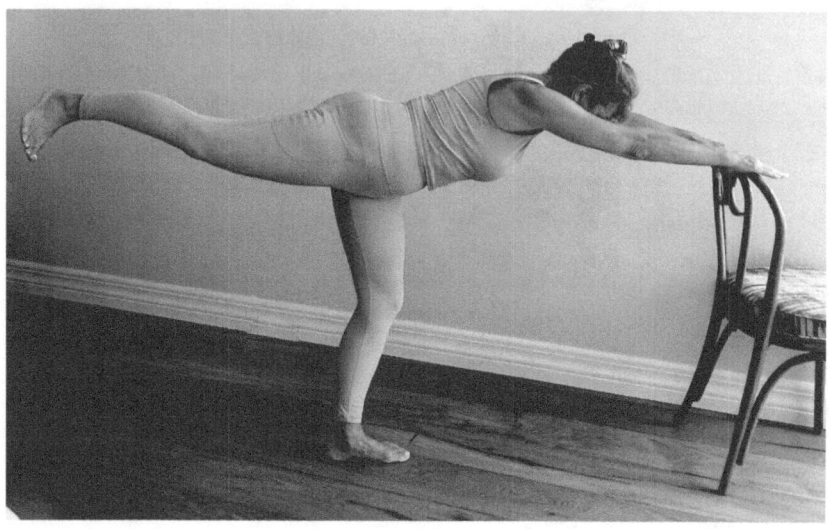

Warrior III Pose Step 4

1. Begin standing behind the back of the chair <u>with the chair's seat against a wall to ensure the chair doesn't slip</u>.
2. Step back from the chair about 2 feet.
3. Bend forward, keeping the legs and spine straight as you reach forward, and place your hands on the back of the chair.
4. Keep your arms straight as you sweep your right leg behind you, creating a straight line from your arms down your back to your flexed foot.
5. Hold this pose for 5 breaths, breathing steadily as you engage the core and relax the shoulders. Keep a slight bend in the knee you are balancing upon.
6. Repeat this posture with your left leg for 5 breaths.

REVERSE WARRIOR III

Open the chest and stretch the spine.

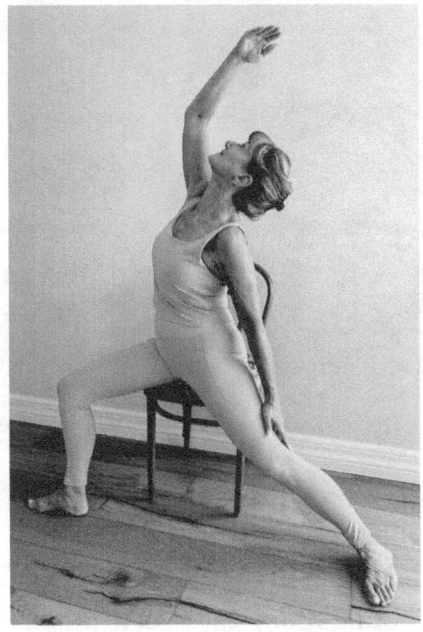

Reverse Warrior III Step 2

1. Begin seated with a tall spine. Rotate your right foot to the right, ensuring your foot is flat on the floor. Extend your left leg straight to the left side with your foot flat on the ground and pointing forward.
2. Align the heel of your front foot with the arch of your back foot.
3. Place your left hand on your left thigh while reaching the right arm up and over your head as far as is comfortable.
4. Allow your gaze to look up into your outstretched palm.
5. Hold this pose to the count of 5.
6. Slowly lower your arm and switch the positions of the legs, repeating this pose to stretch the other side of the body.

HIGH LUNGE TWIST

Open the hips while stretching the spine.

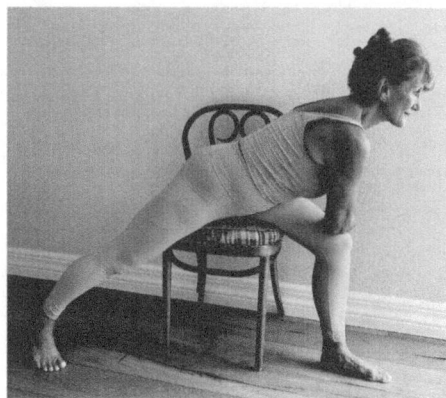
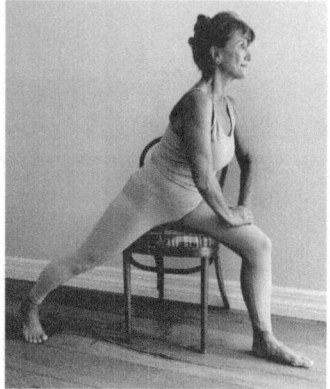

High Lunge Twist Step 4   *High Lunge Twist Modification*

1. Begin seated on the edge of your chair.
2. Swing your left leg to the left so that you are facing the left side while pivoting your right leg down so that the top of your thigh is on the chair seat and your right foot is facing the chair.
3. Ensure that your left foot is flat on the ground while the right foot can be on the ball of your foot.
   Modification- Do not rotate as far for a gentler hip stretch, placing both hands on your knee.
4. Twist the body, bringing the right elbow to the left knee and holding onto the back of the chair.
5. Hold for a count of 5-10.
6. Repeat this pose facing the opposite direction with the right leg forward.

EAGLE ARCH

Deep stretch in the hips and length in the spine.

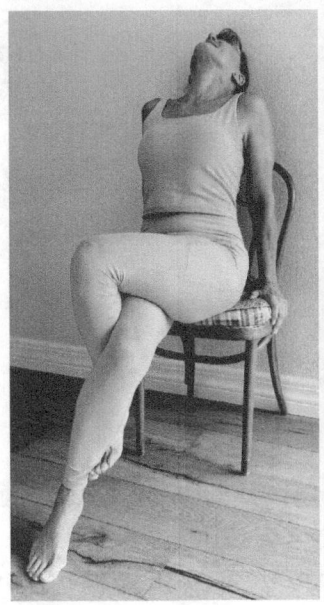 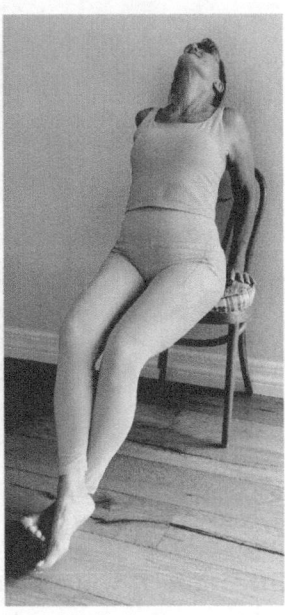

Eagle Arch Step 3   *Eagle Arch Modification*

1. Begin seated on the edge of your chair. Stabilize yourself by gripping the chair seat with your arms.
2. Cross your left leg over your right leg and tuck your left foot behind your right calf, coming into Eagle legs. **Modification**- For a more accessible stretch on your knees and hips, cross your ankles.
3. Place your hands behind you on the chair seat as you arch your chest towards the ceiling and round your back, looking up at the ceiling.
4. Hold for the count of 5 breaths.
5. Repeat on the other side by crossing your right leg over the left.

PLANK PUSH UPS

Tone the core and strengthen the arms.

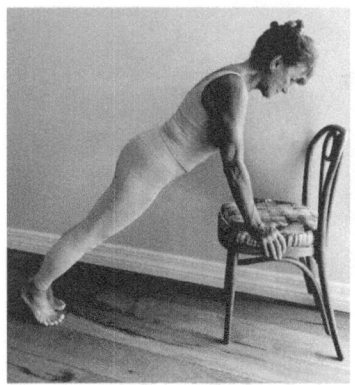 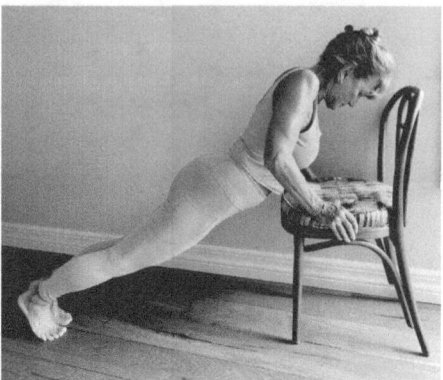

Plank Push Ups Step 3　　　　*Plank Push Ups Step 4*

1. Begin by standing in front of your chair. <u>Brace the chair against a wall so the chair does not slide</u>.
   Modification- If you need a more accessible stretch on your shoulders, perform this posture standing behind the back of your chair.
2. Lean down so both hands are gripping the edge of your chair seat.
3. Step back from the chair so you are on the balls of your feet, forming a straight line from your neck down your spine to your feet. Engage your core.
4. Inhale as you slowly lower your chest to the seat of your chair.
5. Exhale and push yourself away from the chair, tightening your abs as you straighten your arms.
6. Continue for 5 repetitions.

SIDE PLANK

Improve balance and strengthen core and arms.

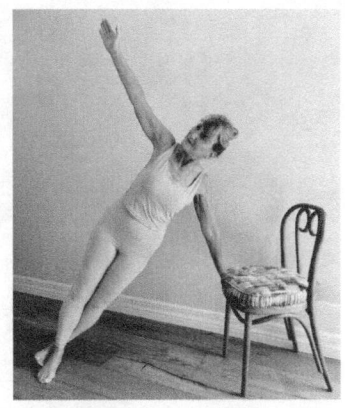

Side Plank Step 4

1. Begin standing in front of the seat of your chair. <u>Brace the back of the chair against the wall so it doesn't slip out from under you</u>.
2. Bend down and place your hands on the chair seat with your fingers spread and pointing to the back of the chair.
   Modification- If you experience pain in your wrist or shoulder, try this pose on the back of the chair instead so there is less pressure on your wrists.
3. Step your feet away from the chair so that you come into a plank pose on the balls of your feet, with your body in a continuous line from your head to your feet. Keep your spine straight and your core engaged.
4. Lift your right arm and extend it toward the ceiling. Rotate your body so that you come onto the side of your left foot. Cross your right foot in front of the left to stabilize your body and balance on your left hand.
5. Hold for the count of 5, keeping your breathing even and controlled.
6. Slowly come out of the pose by lowering the right arm and stepping towards the chair before repeating this pose on the other side of the body.
7. Repeat again on each side of the body.

EXTENDED LEG POSE

Flexibility in the legs while stretching the shoulders.

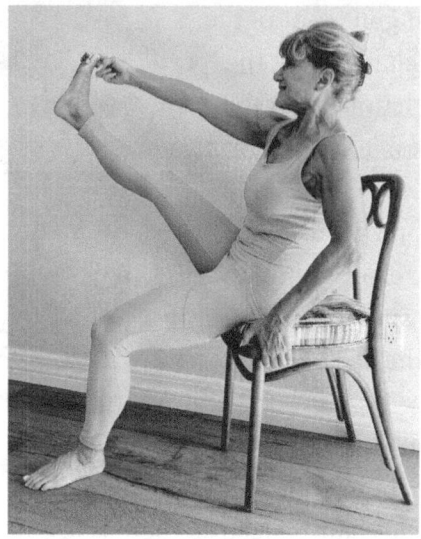

Extended Leg Pose Step 3

1. Begin seated in your chair with a tall spine and your feet flat.
2. Inhale and lift your right foot off the ground, bringing your knee towards your chest.
3. Interlace your pointer and middle fingers of your right hand around your right big toe, and extend your leg forward, straightening it the best you can.
4. Hold the pose to the count of 5, keeping your breathing even and slow.
5. Repeat this exercise with the left leg.

FIVE TIBETAN RITES

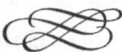

LONGEVITY POSES

> *"Exercise is a celebration for what the body can do, not a punishment for what you ate."*
>
> — *KEVIN NG*

Yoga has positively impacted my life as an engaging form of movement. I am so grateful for how widespread this exercise has become internationally. Another practice, although less well known, also offers a simple and effective way to achieve balance in body and mind and celebrate the incredible vessel we get to use! These are The Five Tibetan Rites. The Five Tibetan Rites is a similar form of exercise to Yoga but specifically focuses on healing and rejuvenating the endocrine system and slowing the aging process through improved organ function and increased vitality. These once-secret ancient exercises have been practiced for over 2,500 years. They focus on clearing and healing the energy centers in the body, also known as the chakras. The seven energy centers are located throughout the body's meridian and determine the body's energetic balance. (Witt, 2024)

The benefits of the Five Tibetan Rites are extensive. By practicing these exercises regularly, individuals can experience improved physical strength, flexibility, and mental clarity. My mother, Leslie, who has been practicing these rites for over 13 years, reports feeling a significant improvement in her physical and psychological well-being. Leslie claims that the Tibetan Rites have predominately increased strength in her core, as well as provide a profound sense of balance and resilience throughout her body. The Five Tibetan Rites are also known to enhance endurance, energy levels, and overall health. (Kurus, 2001)

These poses have been chosen to be the five most effective daily exercises. They are easy to remember and simple to perform, with variations for each pose. In this book, we have adapted the variations for use with the chair for people of any ability to access these ancient postures. These Rites are traditionally repeated 21 times each. Start at 5 repetitions and increase as you feel able. Take time with each exercise and listen to your body. If you experience any health concerns, try a variation on the pose or skip those that may aggravate any health issues.

SPINNING POSE

Improves posture and proprioception, ensures your body's ability to balance naturally, and gets the energy vortexes in the body spinning in the right direction.

Beginner Spinning Pose

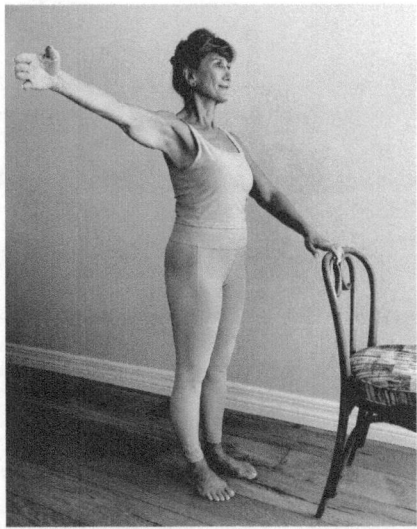

Beginner Spinning Pose Step 4

1. Stand tall behind the chair with your hands balancing on the back.
2. Extend your arms to either side of your body at shoulder height with your palms facing down.
3. Turn the body to the right, keeping the arms extended as you pivot in place, turning in a circle so you are again facing the back of the chair.
4. You can utilize the chair as a support throughout the pose or as needed to ensure you stay balanced as you rotate slowly to the right.
5. Keep your eyes focused on one spot on the wall so that when you turn, your head looks at that focal point as much as possible. Focusing your eyes will help you from getting dizzy.
6. Rotate as many times as you feel comfortable. Start at 5 rotations and work your way up to 21.

Advanced Spinning Pose

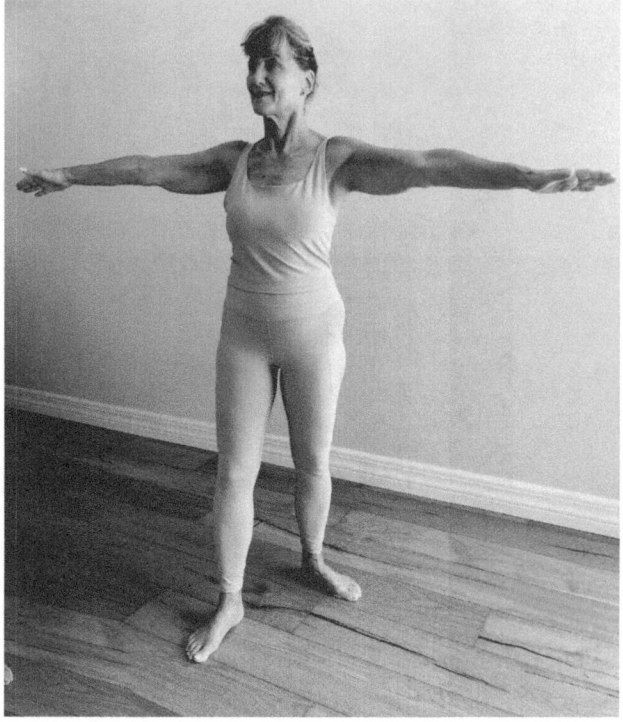

Advanced Spinning Pose Step 3

1. Stand tall with arms outstretched to either side of your body at shoulder height and your palms facing down.
2. Begin turning slowly in a circle to the right. Staying in the same location on the floor as you turn.
3. Keep your eyes focused on one spot on the wall so that when you turn, your head looks at that focal point as much as possible. Focusing your eyes will help you from getting dizzy.
4. Rotate as many times as you feel comfortable. Start at 5 rotations and work your way up to 21.

LEG RAISE

Brings strength to the core and throughout the legs while improving balance.

Beginner Leg Raise

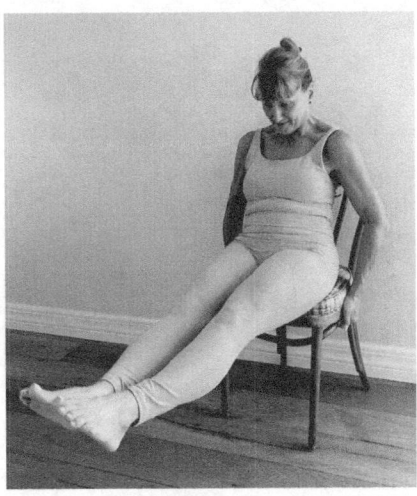

Beginner Leg Raise Step 4

1. Begin seated on the edge of your chair with your feet flat on the ground and your hands gripping the sides of your seat.
2. Lean back in your chair so your back rests on the back of your chair.
3. Extend your legs out, creating a straight line from your feet to your head.
4. Inhale while flexing your feet and lifting your legs off the ground, engaging your core. Keep your breathing even. At the same time tuck your chin towards your chest.
5. Exhale and release your legs back down to the ground while stretching your neck back.
6. Repeat this pose 5 times, working your way up to 21.

Advanced Leg Raise

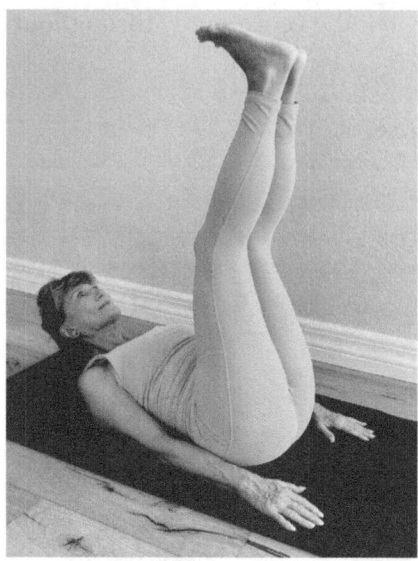

Advanced Leg Raise Step 4

1. Begin lying flat on your back on a yoga mat or rug with your legs together and feet flexed.
2. Extend your hands alongside your sides with your palms flat on the ground.
3. Breathe in as you raise your head and tuck your chin towards your chest.
4. At the same time, lift your legs without bending your knees, bringing your legs over your body and towards your head.
5. Exhale as you slowly lower your legs and head to the floor, relaxing your muscles as your body comes to rest.
6. Repeat this exercise 5 times and work your way up to 21 repetitions.

BACKBEND POSE

Create flexibility and elasticity in the spine while improving posture and balance.

Beginner Backbend Pose

1. Begin seated on the edge of your chair with feet flat on the floor and shoulder-width apart. Place your hands behind you on the seat of the chair.
2. Inhale as you tilt your chin to look down at your lap, stretching the back of your shoulders and neck.
3. Exhale as you tilt your head to look at the ceiling, transferring your weight to your hands as you stretch the whole spine.
4. Inhale as you incline the head forward, bringing the chin to the chest.

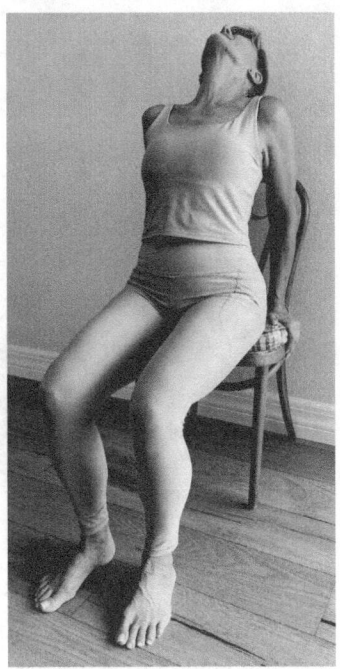

Beginner Backbend Pose Step 3

5. Continue this stretch for 5 repetitions and work your way up to 21 backbends.

Advanced Backbend Pose

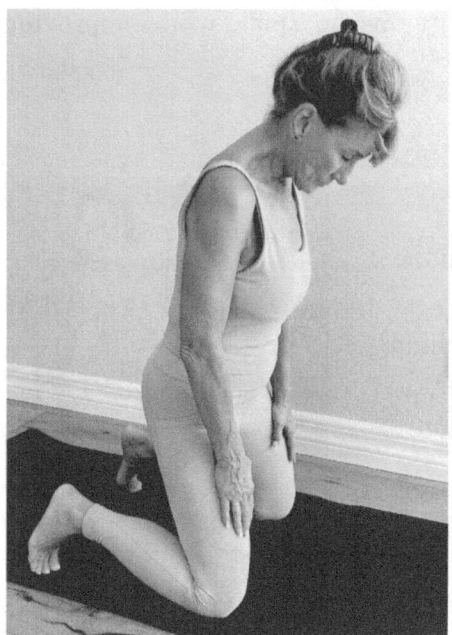 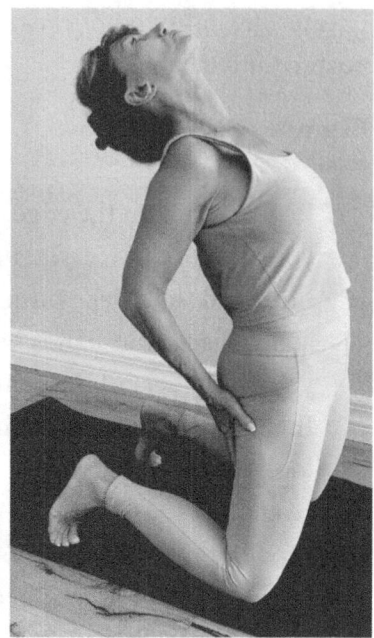

Advanced Backbend Step 2   *Advanced Backbend Step 3*

1. Begin kneeling on your yoga mat or a carpet with your spine tall and your hands braced on your thighs. Your toes are curled under to stabilize the body.
2. Inhale as you incline your chin down to your chest.
3. Exhale as you tilt your head back to look up at the ceiling, arching your spine as you raise your chest towards the ceiling, supported by moving your hands to the backs of your thighs.
4. Repeat this backbend 5 times, working up to 21 repetitions.

TABLETOP POSE

Strengthen the arms and shoulders and challenge balance in the core and legs.

Beginner Tabletop Pose

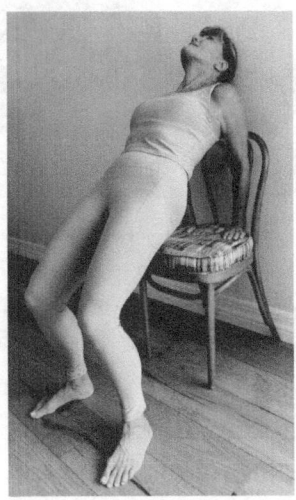

Beginner Tabletop Step 3

1. Begin seated on the edge of your chair with your feet flat on the floor and shoulder-width apart. Place your hands behind you on the seat of the chair.
2. On the inhale, incline your head towards your chin.
3. On the exhale, tilt your head back, shifting your weight onto your hands as you raise your hips towards the ceiling, bending your knees.
4. Slowly lower your hips back into the chair and rest the body before repeating.
5. Continue this exercise for the count of 5, working up to 21 repetitions.

Advanced Tabletop Pose

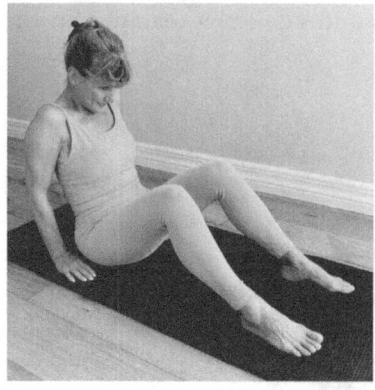

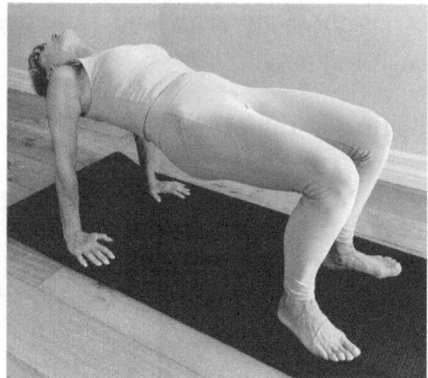

Advanced Tabletop Step 3   *Advanced Tabletop Step 4*

1. Begin seated on your yoga mat or a carpet with your spine tall and your knees bent.
2. Place your palms face down and fingers facing forward on either side of your torso to brace your body.
3. On the inhale, incline your head towards your chin.
4. On the exhale, tilt your head back, raising your body so that your hips become level with your shoulders. Keep your arms straight.
5. Slowly lower your hips back down towards the floor and rest the body.
6. Repeat this exercise 5 times, working up to 21 repetitions.

PENDULUM POSE

Strengthening the spine and shoulders, creating flexibility and balance in the whole body.

Beginner Pendulum Pose

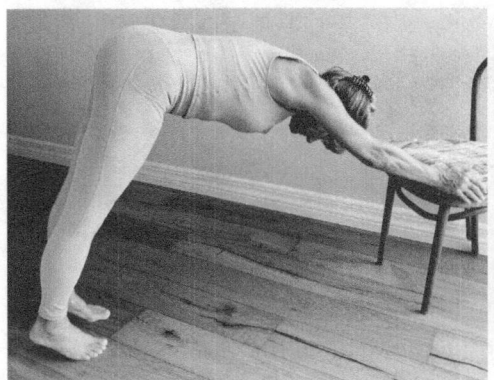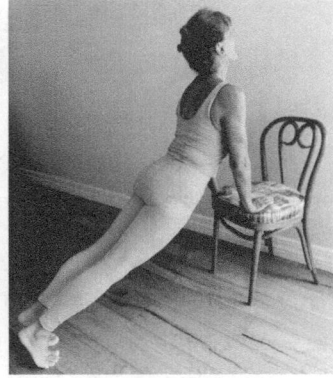

Beginner Pendulum Step 3 *Beginner Pendulum Step 4*

1. Begin standing in front of your chair, facing the chair's seat. <u>Push the back of the chair against the wall to stabilize the chair.</u>
2. Bend down and place your hands on the seat of the chair.
3. Inhale as you step back, bringing your head between your arms and lifting your hips to the sky. Keep arms and spine straight.
4. Exhale as you drop your hips down to the floor, lifting your chest and head up to the sky.
5. Repeat this exercise 5 times, working up to 21 repetitions.

Advanced Pendulum Pose

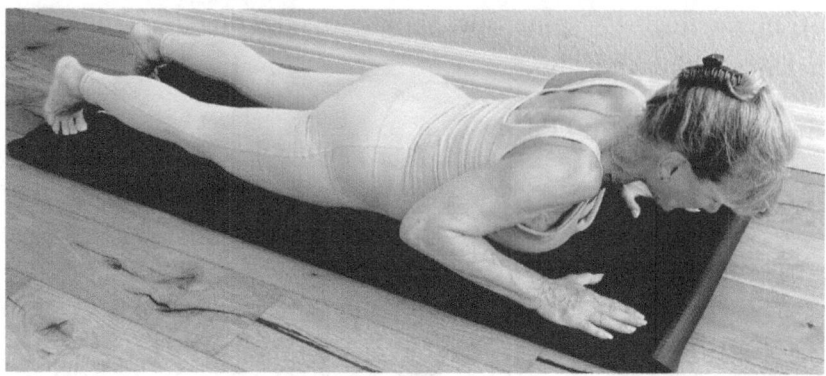

Advanced Pendulum Step 1

1. Begin laying face down on your yoga mat or carpet with your palms face down on either side of the chest. Your toes curled under and flexed.
2. Inhale and lift the hips towards the ceiling, bringing your head between your arms, keeping the arms and spine straight and the body in a "V" shape, like downward dog pose.
3. Exhale and lower the hips, arching the spine and tilting the head backward towards the sky so you come into an upward dog pose. Repeat this exercise 5 times, working up to 21 repetitions.

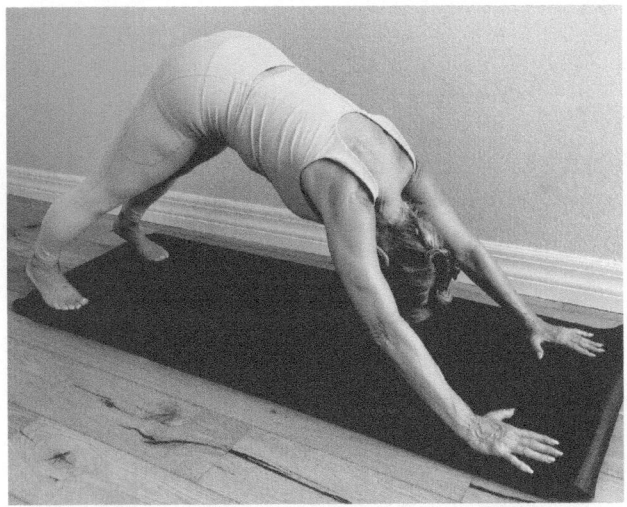

Advanced Pendulum Step 2

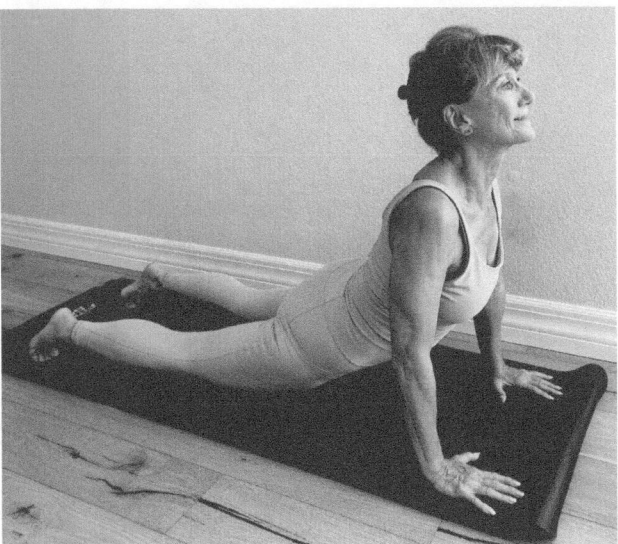

Advanced Pendulum Step 3

COOL DOWN

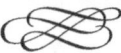

NURTURING YOUR BODY, CALMING YOUR MIND

"Go confidently in the direction of your dreams. Live the life you have imagined, and you will meet with success."

— *HENRY DAVID THOREAU*

After 40 years of teaching yoga, Connie Dennison still taught at age 100. She is considered one of the oldest living yoga teachers, with some of her students attending her classes for over 30 years. Many believe she is a walking advertisement for the benefits of Yoga. She claims that the real benefits of Yoga are that it has kept her mobile, and even able to drive her car into her 90s. She says, "I'm sure Yoga is what kept me young. I'd be in a wheelchair if it weren't for Yoga. If you don't use it, you lose it." Connie recounts injuring herself, resulting in a slipped disk, and through Yoga, healing her body and recovering from the injury. Even though Connie Dennison passed away at the age of 102, she continues to inspire the devotion to health and wellness that we can seek at any age. (Lawrie, 2015)

THE SLOW STRETCHES: CREATING CLOSURE

As we near the end of our Chair Yoga routine, it's essential to transition gracefully from movement to stillness, from effort to ease. This chapter will explore the importance of a gentle and soothing cool-down sequence. The cool-down offers an opportunity to release tension and cultivate calm relaxation in both body and mind.

Cooling down after physical activity is crucial for seniors to help prevent injury, reduce muscle soreness, and promote recovery. It also provides a space for reflection, integration, and gratitude, allowing you to honor your efforts during your practice and acknowledge your body's resilience.

After engaging in physical activity, your muscles may feel tight or fatigued. The cool-down allows your muscles to slowly relax and recover, reducing the risk of stiffness or soreness. These exercises also help gradually lower your heart rate and blood pressure, promoting cardiovascular health and preventing dizziness or lightheadedness.

The cool-down phase lets you shift your focus inward, cultivating a sense of calm. It allows you to transition from the external world to inner peace.

SPINE STRETCH

Elongate the spine and stretch the shoulder, loosening the muscles in the arms.

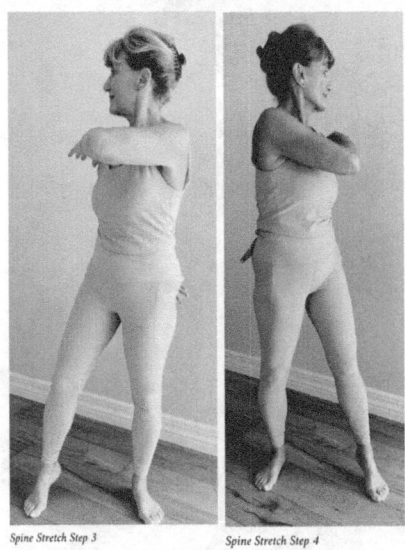

Spine Stretch Step 3   Spine Stretch Step 4

1. Stand tall with your feet shoulder-width apart.
2. Extend your arms to either side of your body at shoulder height with your palms facing down.
3. Swing your arms to the right, allowing your left hand to gently slap your right shoulder and your right hand to slap your lower back.
4. Allow your spine and legs to follow the movement of your arms without lifting your feet off the ground. Your heels may lift from the floor slightly.
5. Turn to the left, with your torso and arms following. Keep your head turning in the direction of your arms.
6. Continue for 10 repetitions.

HAMSTRING CURL

Stretch out the muscles of the calves.

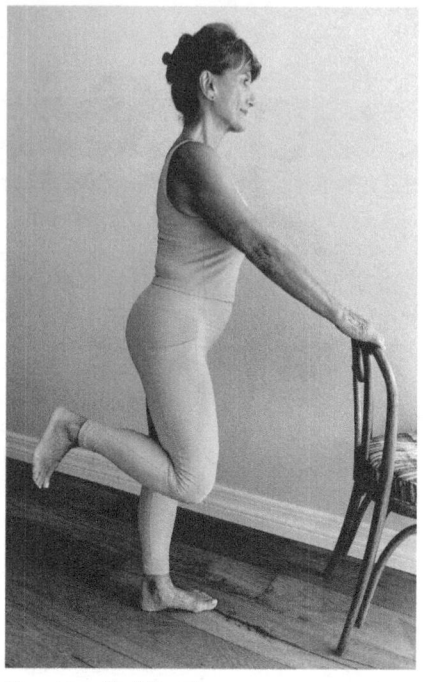

Hamstring Curl Step 2

1. Begin by standing behind the chair holding onto the backrest with your feet shoulder-width apart.
2. As you inhale, keep your thigh and knee still as you slowly raise the heel of the right foot behind you as high as possible.
3. Slowly lower your right leg down with control.
4. Continue for 5 total repetitions.
5. Repeat with the left hamstring for 5 repetitions.

KNEE HOLDS

Stretch the muscles in the hips and back.

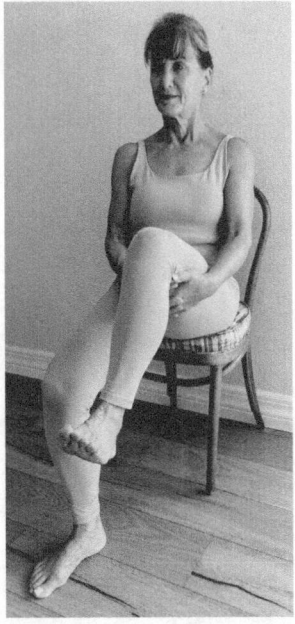

Knee Holds Step 2

1. Start by sitting on the edge of the seat of your chair.
2. Reach down and interlock your fingers under the thigh of your left leg.
3. Keep your back straight as you pull up on your thigh, rotating the knee in a circular motion while flexing the left foot.
4. Continue for the count of 5.
5. Repeat with the right leg.

SHOULDER ROLLS

Relax the muscles in the shoulders and neck.

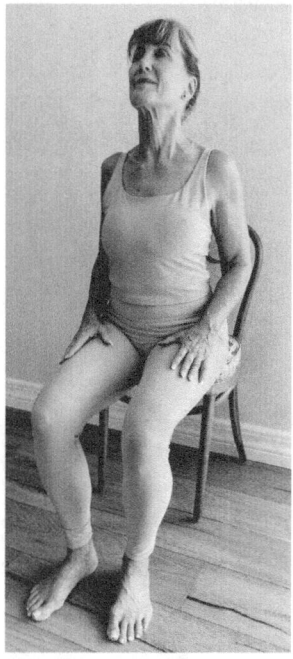

Shoulder Rolls Step 3

1. Begin seated with your spine straight and arms relaxed on your thighs.
2. Inhale as you raise your shoulders towards your ears.
3. Exhale as you roll your shoulders back and down.
4. Continue for the count of 10, breathing evenly through the rolls.

ANKLE ROLLS

Release tension in the legs, ankles, and feet.

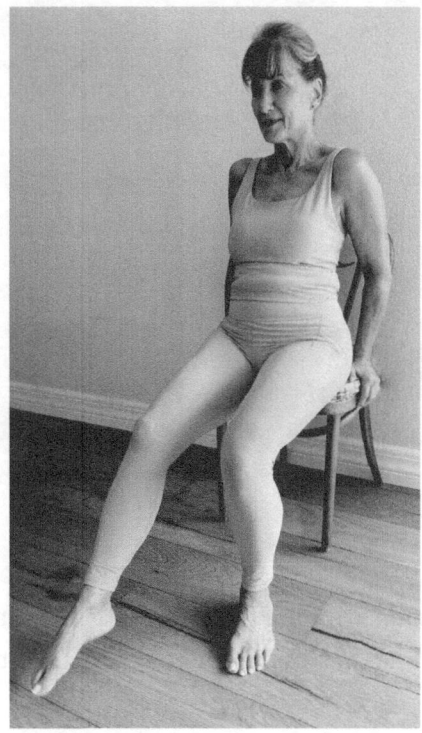

Ankle Rolls Step 2

1. Begin seated on the chair with your hands holding the edges of your chair seat and your feet shoulder-width apart.
2. Lift your right foot and rotate the ankle clockwise for the count of 3.
3. Rotate the right foot in a counterclockwise direction for the count of 3.
4. Repeat with your left foot.

LEG EXTENDERS

Release tension in the calves and thighs, stretching out the back of the knee.

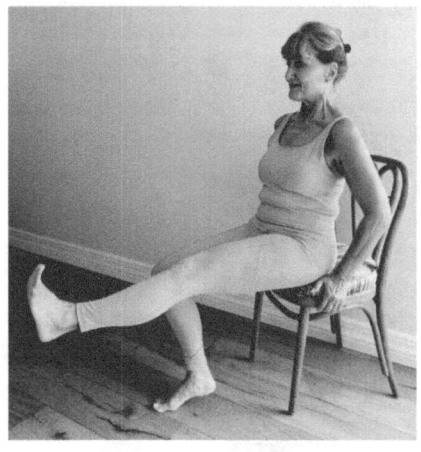 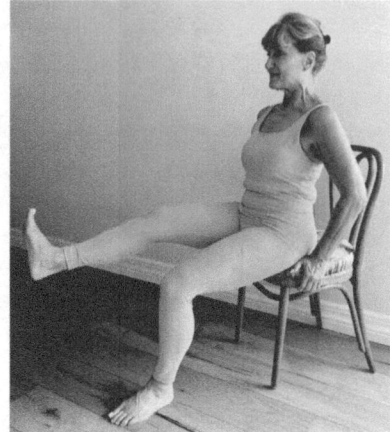

Leg Extenders Step 2   *Leg Extenders Step 4*

1. Begin seated on the edge of your chair with your spine tall and your hands gripping the edges of the chair seat.
2. Lift your left leg in front of you to knee height, keeping the foot flexed.
3. Slowly lower your foot down to the ground.
4. Lift your right leg in front of you to knee height, keeping the foot flexed. Slowly lower your foot down to the ground.
5. Repeat these exercises 5 times in total.

PRAYER TWIST

Stretch out the spine.

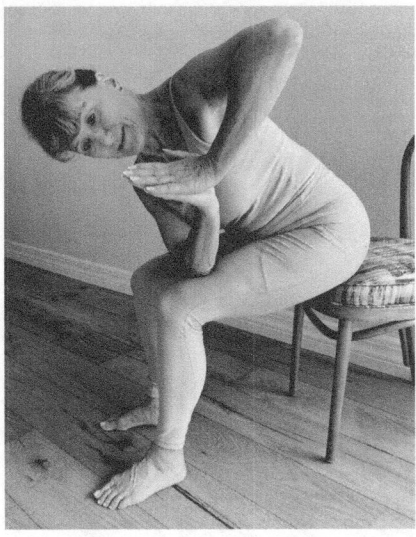

Prayer Twist Step 3

1. Begin seated on the chair with both feet shoulder-width apart and flat on the ground.
2. Bring the palms of your hands together in front of your heart.
3. Rotate to the left, bringing your right elbow down to your left knee.
4. Hold for the count of 5.
5. Repeat on the other side, bringing your left elbow to your right knee.

TRICEPS STRETCH

Stretch the shoulders and arms and create length in the spine.

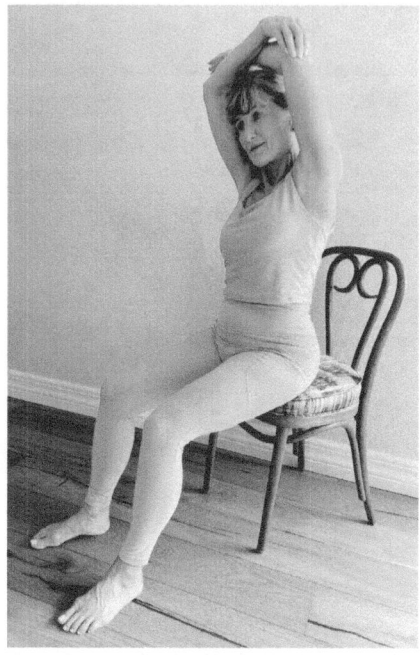

Triceps Stretch Step 2

1. Begin seated in your chair with your feet shoulder-width apart and your shoulders relaxed.
2. Reach your arms over your head and grasp your left elbow with your right hand, gently pulling to the right.
3. Hold for the count of 5.
4. Repeat on the other side, grasping your right elbow with your left hand and gently pulling to the left.
5. Hold for the count of 5.

CONCLUSION

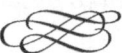

KEEPING THE MOMENTUM

> *"Take Pride in how far you have come and have faith in how far you can go."*
>
> — *MICHAEL JOSEPHSON*

Keeping up with your physical goals can be challenging, but it is gratifying to realize your power. Feeling confident in your body makes you feel strong, enhancing your mind, which makes you want to exercise more, ultimately making you feel even better. This courage creates a positive spiral that ripples out around you, influencing not only your physical well-being but also your mental and emotional health.

Taking care of your body generates feel-good endorphins that leave a lasting impression on your life, enhancing your mood and giving you confidence. This dedication often attracts other people who also prioritize their health. This community of like-minded individuals can provide support, encouragement, and motivation, further enhancing your wellness journey.

Physical activity can burn off harmful calories, reducing the risk of various health issues more effectively than a sedentary lifestyle. Moving our bodies through Chair Yoga serves as a detox, rejuvenating our bodies by promoting blood flow and creating new muscle memory for faster recovery. This gentle yet effective exercise accommodates different mobility levels while providing a robust workout, leaving room to excel forward as well.

Incorporating Chair Yoga into your routine supports physical health and boosts mental clarity and emotional resilience. The mindful movements and breathwork involved in Yoga can reduce stress, improve focus, and elevate mood. As you continue to practice, you will likely sleep better, feel more energetic, and have a greater sense of well-being.

Remember, the journey to maintaining and improving your health is ongoing and unique to everyone. Celebrate your progress, no matter how small, and remain patient and compassionate with yourself.

In conclusion, Chair Yoga offers seniors a safe, accessible, and highly effective way to stay active and healthy. Committing to regular practice can enhance your physical fitness, mental acuity, and emotional well-being, paving the way for a vibrant and fulfilling life. Embrace the power of movement, and let it transform you from the inside out.

THE 21-DAY CHAIR YOGA CHALLENGE

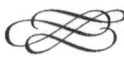

TRANSFORM YOUR BODY, MIND, AND SPIRIT

Welcome to the 21-Day Chair Yoga Challenge—a transformative journey designed to inspire and motivate our desire to improve our well-being. Each workout day is unique, utilizing the exercises featured in this book. These exercises are tailored to bring life to your practice in an inspiring way, creating a realistic space for growth and vitality. A comprehensive way to integrate Chair Yoga practices into your routine, this Challenge is curated to support you on your path to radiant health.

The 21-day-long Challenge invites you to commit to your self-care and embark on a journey of renewal. Over 21 days, you will explore a variety of Chair Yoga practices, including gentle stretches, strengthening exercises, mindfulness techniques, and relaxation practices. Each day offers a new opportunity to connect with yourself, cultivate mindfulness, and embrace the transformative power of Yoga.

As you embark on this journey, remember that the most crucial aspect of the Challenge is not perfection but commitment. Whether you're new to Yoga or a seasoned practitioner, approach each day with an open heart and a willingness to explore the depths of your body, mind, and spirit. Trust in the process, honor your unique needs and limitations, and celebrate the progress you make throughout the Challenge.

INTENTIONAL JOURNEY: ROAD TO SUCCESS

Before embarking on the 21-Day Chair Yoga Challenge, take a moment to set intentions for your practice. Consider what you hope to gain from this journey—weight loss, increased flexibility, reduced stress, improved strength, or simply a sense of peace and well-being. Set your intentions with clarity and compassion.

The 21-Day Chair Yoga Challenge is structured to provide you with a diverse array of practices to support your physical, mental, and emotional well-being. Each day, you will engage in a guided Chair Yoga practice tailored to address specific aspects of your well-being, such as flexibility, strength, balance, or relaxation. These practices will range in length from 5 to 15 minutes a day, making them accessible and manageable for seniors with busy schedules.

Alongside your Chair Yoga poses will be mindfulness breathing techniques to help calm your mind, reduce stress, and cultivate present-moment awareness. Completing each day with breath-work will complement your yoga practice and deepen your connection to yourself.

At the end of each day, reflect on your experience and insights gained from the day's practice. The reflection prompts provided will encourage you to cultivate self-awareness and gratitude as you navigate the challenges and joys of the 21-Day Chair Yoga journey.

What to Expect Week by Week

The Challenge will begin with simple beginner poses that focus on posture and balance in the first week, anchoring our bodies into a routine that is nourishing and attainable with quick 5 minutes sessions.

As we move into the second week, we will explore our body's flexibility and stability by incorporating intermediate poses into our daily practice. These poses will focus on gaining muscle, building joint resilience, and increasing our energy with endorphin-building exercises.

Progressing into the third week will be a mastery of your body and mind as we incorporate all we have learned into a daily practice that brings strength, empowerment, and joy to our day. We will celebrate our progress and all we have achieved through reflection and integration of postures that challenge and invite new sensations and abilities.

WEEK 1: FOUNDATIONS

Welcome to the 21-Day Chair Yoga Challenge, an attainable way to bring exercise into your routine with daily guided exercises and meditations.

Day 1: Gentle Flow

1. Prayer Pose
2. Shoulder Rotations
3. Cat-Cow Pose
4. Marching Pose
5. Toe Heel Raises
6. Sphinx Pose

7. Back Stretch
8. Hip Circles
9. Ankle Rolls
10. Diaphragmatic Breathing

Reflection: How can I honor that which is sacred in my life? I deserve the time to step into my power.

Day 2: Mindfulness Made

1. Seated Mountain Pose
2. Neck Rotations
3. Arm Reach
4. Side Twist
5. Crescent Moon Pose
6. Warrior I Pose
7. Chair Lunge
8. Hamstring Curl
9. Prayer Twist
10. Alternate Nostril Breathing

Reflection: I see only beauty reflected in my heart when I have clear vision.

Day 3: Positive Perception

1. Prayer Pose
2. Shoulder Rotations
3. Cat-Cow
4. Arm Reach
5. Side Bend
6. Forward Fold
7. Side Leg Raises

8. Spine Stretch
9. Triceps Stretch
10. Ujjayi Breathing

Reflection: My positive state of mind draws blessings into my life.

Day 4: Give Joy

1. Seated Mountain Pose
2. Marching Pose
3. Forward Fold
4. Chest Opener
5. Back Stretch
6. Side Leg Raises
7. Standing Knee Taps
8. Chair Lunge
9. Hamstring Curl
10. Sitali Breathing

Reflection: When I cultivate joy and right relationship to all things, my heart is light as a feather.

Day 5: Becoming Balance

1. Prayer Pose
2. Neck Rotations
3. Marching Pose
4. Toe- Heel Raises
5. Side Twist
6. Hip Circles
7. Supported Squats
8. Spine Stretch
9. Knee Holds

10. Bee Breath

Reflection: Listen to the teachings of the great trees. What wisdom of balance do they impart as they weather the storms?

Day 6: Graceful Renewal

1. Shoulder Rotations
2. Marching Pose
3. Forward Fold
4. Crescent Moon Pose
5. Sphinx Pose
6. Spinal Twist with Arm Reach
7. Hip Circles
8. Warrior I Pose
9. Leg Extenders
10. Shavasana

Reflection: Sometimes, old forms and habits must be surrendered for life to be renewed and reborn into higher forms.

Day 7: Boundless Fortitude

1. Seated Mountain Pose
2. Cat–Cow Pose
3. Side Bend Pose
4. Side Twist
5. Sphinx Pose
6. Back Stretch
7. Warrior I Pose
8. Standing Knee Taps
9. Shoulder Rolls
10. Diaphragmatic Breathing

Reflection: Each dawn is a new promise and a new chance to remake my world.

WEEK 2: BUILDING MOMENTUM IN MINDFUL MOVEMENT

You are on track to making a healthy routine with Chair Yoga, enjoy these moments to cherish your body with self-care.

Day 8: Abundance Blossoming

1. Neck Rotations
2. Arm Reach
3. Cobra Pose
4. Eagle Arms
5. Dancers Pose
6. Triangle Pose
7. Downward Dog
8. Upward Plank
9. Knee Holds
10. Alternate Nostril Breathing

Reflection: Today I spend time in a blossoming garden of my own creation and breathe deeply the scents of flowering fruit trees.

Day 9: Attention to Detail

1. Toe Heel Raises
2. Side Bend
3. Pigeon Pose
4. Chair Squats
5. Plank Pose
6. Mountain Climbers Pose

7. Butterfly Pose
8. Warrior II Pose
9. Shoulder Rolls
10. Ujjayi Breathing

Reflection: If I focus on what is most important, the way will be opened for me to move ahead.

Day 10: Faith in the Face of Fire

1. Seated Mountain Pose
2. Cat-Cow Pose
3. Chest Opener
4. Cobra Pose
5. Boat Pose
6. Triangle Pose
7. Chair Pose
8. Upward Plank
9. Ankle Rolls
10. Sitali Breathing

Reflection: How can I continue to strive for my inner beliefs and desires? I believe in myself.

Day 11: Mind Over Matter

1. Prayer Pose
2. Spinal Twist with Arm Reach
3. Supported Squats
4. Eagle Arms
5. Plank Pose
6. Dancers Pose
7. Leg Lifts

8. Butterfly Pose
9. Triceps Stretch
10. Bee Breath

Reflection: I remain ever mindful of the nature of the thoughts I hold, knowing my thoughts create my world.

Day 12: Gratitude is My Attitude

1. Neck Rotations
2. Chest Opener
3. Side Leg Raises
4. Cobra Pose
5. Boat Pose
6. Chair Squats
7. Downward Dog
8. Warrior II Pose
9. Leg Extenders
10. Shavasana

Reflection: I choose to be playful today and face the day with childlike wonder.

Day 13: Dedication is in my routine.

Beginner Tibetan Rites Exploration

1. Shoulder Rotations
2. Spinning Pose
3. Leg Raise
4. Backbend Pose
5. Tabletop Pose
6. Pendulum Pose

7. Pigeon Pose
8. Spine Stretch
9. Prayer Twist
10. Diaphragmatic Breathing

Reflection: Change is all around me, but I stay true to my course and focus on my goals.

Day 14: Strength In Acceptance

1. Arm Reach
2. Crescent Moon Pose
3. Standing Knee Taps
4. Eagle Arms
5. Mountain Climbers
6. Leg Lifts
7. Chair Pose
8. Warrior II Pose
9. Hamstring Curl
10. Alternate Nostril Breathing

Reflection: How can accepting myself change my perception of the world?

WEEK 3: MEETING YOUR GOALS: COMPLETING THE CHALLENGE

Finding the internal power to complete this challenge is an accomplishment showing your personal strength. You can do anything that you set your mind upon.

Day 15: Destined for Greatness

1. Side Bend
2. Spinal Twist with Arm Reach
3. Upward Dog
4. Gate Pose
5. Warrior III
6. Reverse Warrior III
7. High Lunge Twist
8. Eagle Arch
9. Knee Holds
10. Ujjayi Breathing

Reflection: I make the most of the situation I am granted today.

Day 16: Enter the Adventure

1. Toe Heel Raises
2. Chair Lunge
3. Leg Lifts
4. Upward Plank
5. Extended Side Angle
6. 3-Legged Downward Dog
7. Lifted Core Pose
8. Side Plank
9. Shoulder Rolls
10. Sitali Breathing

Reflection: I engage my sense of adventure as I enter the wild and mysterious places within myself.

Day 17: I Lean into Growth

1. Forward Fold
2. Plank Pose
3. Mountain Climbers Pose
4. Gate Pose
5. Low Lunge
6. Reverse Warrior 3 Pose
7. Extended Leg Pose
8. Hamstring Curl
9. Ankle Rolls
10. Bee Breath

Reflection: I remember not to take myself too seriously as I face what the universe provides.

Day 18: Desire for Accomplishment

1. Seated Mountain Pose
2. Side Twist
3. Upward Dog
4. Low Lunge
5. Warrior III
6. Eagle Arch
7. Lifted Core Pose
8. Side Plank
9. Leg Extenders
10. Shavasana

Reflection: My soul longs to create something of beauty; what fuel drives my desires?

Day 19: Nurturing Self Awareness

Advanced Tibetan Rites Exploration

1. Supported Squats
2. Dancers Pose
3. Triangle Pose
4. Adv. Spinning Pose
5. Adv. Leg Raise
6. Adv. Backbend Pose
7. Adv. Tabletop Pose
8. Adv. Pendulum Pose
9. Shoulder Rolls
10. Diaphragmatic Breathing

Reflection: What truth is reflected when I let my inner beauty unfold?

Day 20: Elegant Balance

1. Prayer Pose
2. Chair Squats
3. Downward Dog
4. Butterfly Pose
5. Extended Side Angle
6. 3-Legged Downward Dog
7. High Lunge Twist
8. Extended Leg Pose
9. Triceps Stretch
10. Alternate Nostril Breathing

Reflection: My heart blooms open like a rose when I discover my worth and power.

Day 21: Awakening Purpose

1. Neck Rotations
2. Boat Pose
3. Leg Lifts
4. Chair Pose
5. Upward Dog
6. Warrior III
7. Reverse Warrior III
8. Eagle Arch
9. Prayer Twist
10. Shavasana

Reflection: Each dawn holds a new promise, a new chance to explore my world.

INTEGRATING OUR PRACTICE: THE PATH TOWARDS RADIANT HEALTH

As we conclude our 21-Day Chair Yoga Challenge, let us embrace the journey ahead with open hearts and minds. This Challenge offers a unique opportunity to deepen your connection to yourself, cultivate self-awareness, and unlock the transformative power of Yoga.

Throughout this book, we have explored various gentle, yet potent practices designed to support your physical, mental, and emotional well-being. From foundational postures to advanced sequences, from mindful breathing to deep relaxation, Chair Yoga offers a pathway to radiant health and vitality at any age.

As you integrate the teachings of Chair Yoga into your daily life, may you embrace the wisdom of your body, honoring its unique needs and limitations with kindness and compassion. May you cultivate a sense of gratitude for the miraculous vessel that carries you through this journey of life, and may you find joy and fulfillment in nurturing your body, mind, and spirit through Yoga.

As we come to the end of this book, know that the wisdom and teachings of Yoga will continue to guide and support you on your path to radiant health and well-being. May you continue to embrace the practice with an open heart and an adventurous spirit, knowing that the journey of Yoga is infinite and ever-unfolding.

With deepest gratitude and warmest wishes for your continued journey,

Rachel and Leslie Haduch

Now that you have unlocked the power of Chair Yoga for Seniors, we would love to know about your Chair Yoga journey! Help us by sharing your newfound knowledge and guide other readers to the same transformative experience.

How You Can Keep the Flame Alive:

- **Leave Your Honest Opinion on Amazon:** Your review isn't just words; it's a beacon for other readers, helping them find the information they want. Your passion for Chair Yoga can inspire others to embark on their own journey.
- **Spread the Word:** Share your thoughts on social media or recommend this book to friends and family. Your personal recommendation can spark curiosity and motivate someone to explore the benefits of Chair Yoga.
- **Give the Gift of Knowledge:** Consider gifting a copy to someone you care about. Your gesture might be the push they need to start a positive change in their life.

Remember, **the flame of knowledge** doesn't flicker out when shared; it grows brighter. Thank you for being an integral part of this community and helping keep the flame alive!

Your contribution echoes far beyond these pages, and for that, we are sincerely grateful.

Until we meet again on the path of continued discovery,

~Rachel and Leslie~

REFERENCES

Marching Pose Yoga. (n.d) Tummee. https://www.tummee.com/yoga-poses/ marching-pose

The Yogic Encyclopedia. (2024) Ananda. *https://www.ananda.org/yogapedia/yoga/*

A Brief History of Yoga. (2020, August 6) The Art of Living. https://www.artofliving. org/us-en/yoga/beginners/yoga-history

McGee, Kristin. (2022, November 21) *11 Types of Yoga: A Breakdown of the Major Styles.* Mind Body Green Movement. https://www.mindbodygreen.com/arti cles/the-11-major-types-of-yoga-explained-simply

What is Lakshmi Voelker Chair Yoga? (2022) Lakshmi Voelker Chair Yoga. https:// www.lvchairyoga.com/why-chair-yoga

Jordan, Caroline. (2017, June 9) *You Are Only One Workout Away from a Good Mood.* Thrive Global. https://community.thriveglobal.com/you-are-only-one-work out-away-from-a-good-mood/

Feirereison, Sharon. (2023, October 17) *37 Motivational Exercise Quotes to Get You Through Your Next Workout.* Real Simple. https://www.realsimple.com/health/ fitness-exercise/exercise-quotes

Eve. (2014, February 21) *Take a Seat in Utkatasana, the Yoga Chair: Five-Minute Yoga Challenge.* Five Minute Yoga. https://myfiveminuteyoga.com/5107/take-a-seat-in-utkatasana-the-yoga-chair-five-minute-yoga-challenge/

Buckley, Cat. (2023, July 5) The Ultimate Guide to Yoga for Osteoporosis. AlgaeCal. https://blog.algaecal.com/yoga-for-osteoporosis/

Pro Gym Workout. (2018, October 31) *Incline Mountain Climber On Chair for Ladies.* YouTube. https://www.youtube.com/watch?v=mYBDOL8h0Ao

Queen Street Studio. (2023, July 12) Best Chair Yoga Poses. YouTube. https://www. youtube.com/watch?v=71Yq1FKPpnY

About Lakshmi Voelker, The Creator of Chair Yoga. (2022) Lakshmi Voelker Chair Yoga. https://www.lvchairyoga.com/about-lakshmi-voelker

Lynch, Tao-Porchon. (2021, September 2) *Tao Porchon-Lynch Shares 7 Secrets to Aging Gracefully.* Yoga Journal. https://www.yogajournal.com/lifestyle/tao-porchon-lynch-shares-7-secrets-to-aging-gracefully/

About Tao. (2017) Tao Porchon-Lynch. https://www.taoporchon-lynch.com/ about.html

My Story. (2024) Vivian Stancil Olympian Foundation. https://vivianstan cilolympianfoundation.org/

Levy, Jessica. (2021, June 3) *Blindness and Fear Didn't Stop this Woman from Becoming a Star Swimmer.* USA Today. https://www.usatoday.com/story/sponsor-story/humana/2021/06/03/blindness-and-fear-didnt-stop-woman-becoming-star-swimmer/7505208002/

Everheart, Denise. (2024) *The Beginner's Guide to Pranayama: Yoga Breathing Exercises.* The Art of Living. https://www.artofliving.org/us-en/breathwork/pranayama/breathing-exercises

Three-Part Breath (Dirgha Pranayama) Meaning, Steps and Benefits. (2023) Prana Sutra. https://www.prana-sutra.com/post/three-part-breath-dirgha-pranayama-yoga-technique

Cronkleton, Emily. (2023, May 24) *What are the Benefits and Risks of Alternate Nostril Breathing?* Healthline. https://www.healthline.com/health/alternate-nostril-breathing

EkhartYoga. (2024) *A Guide to Ujjayi Breath.* Ekhart Yoga. https://www.ekhartyoga.com/articles/practice/a-guide-to-ujjayi-breath

Ekhart, Esther. (2024) *Cool Down with Sitali Pranayama.* Ekhart Yoga. https://www.ekhartyoga.com/articles/practice/cool-down-with-sitali-pranayama

Husseiny, Richard. (2022, November 28) *Brahmari Pranayama: How To, Benefits, and Uses.* Yogajala. https://yogajala.com/bhramari-pranayama/

Bhramari Pranayama Benefits and How to do the Humming Bee Breath in Yoga. (2023) Prana Sutra. https://www.prana-sutra.com/post/bhramari-pranayama-steps-benefits

Corpse Shavasana. (2023) Yoga Basics. https://www.yogabasics.com/asana/corpse/

Sienra, Regina. (2023, January 17) *97-Year-Old Gymnast Inspires the World with her Incredible Abilities.* My Modern Met. https://mymodernmet.com/johanna-quaas-gymnast/

Natale, Nicol. (2020, December 23) *Watch the World's Oldest Gymnast Crush a Seriously Impressive Routine in Viral Video.* The Washington Post. https://www.prevention.com/fitness/a35056966/johanna-quaas-gymnastics-video-twitter/

Why Good Posture Matters. (2017, January 24) Harvard Health Publishing. https://www.health.harvard.edu/staying-healthy/why-good-posture-matters

Sampson, JoAnne. (2022) *Inspiring Story of Youthful Senior Athlete.* JoAnne Still Got Game. https://joannstillgotgame.com/

Hallandale Beach Resident Leads the Way. (2022, May 18) South Florida Sun Times. https://www.southfloridasuntimes.com/news/hallandale-beach-resident-leads-the-way%3A-at-the-2022-national-senior-games-in-fort-lauderdale

Levy, Jessica. (2021, June 17) *Four Knee Replacement Surgeries Didn't Slow Down this Senior Athlete.* USA Today. https://www.usatoday.com/story/sponsor-story/humana/2021/06/17/four-knee-replacement-surgeries-didnt-slow-down-senior-athlete/7732180002/

Jeraci, Allison Ray. (n.d.) *Use a Chair to Get More Out of Warrior II.* Yoga International. https://yogainternational.com/article/view/use-a-chair-to-get-more-out-of-warrior-ii/#Variation%202:%20Seated%20on%20A%20Chair

Blount, Rachel. (2015, July 8) *National Senior Games athlete discovers 'there is fun after 70'.* Star Tribune. https://www.startribune.com/national-senior-games-athlete-discovers-there-is-fun-after-70/312700681/?refresh=true

Ng, Kevin. (2018, February 18) *Exercise is a Celebration of What the Body Can Do, not a Punishment for What you Ate.* Kevin Ng Yoga and Mindfulness. https://www.kevinngyoga.com/blog/2018/2/28/exercise-is

Kurus, Mary. (2001) *The Five Tibetan Rites: Exercises for Healing, Rejuvenation, and Longevity.* MK Projects. http://www.mkprojects.com/pf_TibetanRites.htm

Witt, Carolinda. (2024) *5 Tibetan Rites: Benefits, History and Step-by-Step Guide.* T5T – The Five Tibetans. https://t5t.com/5-tibetan-rites#:

Frederick, Bridget. (2021, August 27) *Strengthening Pose of the Week: Upward Facing Dog Pose.* Yoga for Times of Change. https://www.yogafortimesofchange.com/strengthening-pose-of-the-week-upward-facing-dog-pose/

YJ Editors. (2022, December 9) *Extended Side Angle Pose: How to Practice Utthita Parsvakonasana.* Yoga Journal. https://www.yogajournal.com/poses/extended-side-angle-pose-2/

Open Door Yoga. (2022, January 11) *20 Minute Yoga – Yoga for Chair – Gate Pose Flow.* YouTube. https://www.youtube.com/watch?v=vx7iDsbqr6c

YJ Editors. (2022, December 9) *Warrior 3 Pose: How to Practice Virabhadrasana III.* Yoga Journal. https://www.yogajournal.com/poses/warrior-iii-pose/

Rasmussen, Rebecca. (n.d.) *9 Soothing Chair Stretches to Release Hip Pain.* Paleo Hacks. https://blog.paleohacks.com/chair-stretches-release-hip-pain/

The Henry D. Thoreau Mis-Quotation Page. (n.d.) The Waldon Woods Project. https://www.walden.org/what-we-do/library/thoreau/mis-quotations/

Hamstring Curls. (n.d.) Enhance Therapy. https://enhancetherapy.com/portfolio/hamstring-curls/

Lawrie, Alexander. (2015, April 6) *Yoga Teacher to Teach Again After She Turns 100.* The Scotsman. https://www.scotsman.com/news/yoga-teacher-to-teach-again-after-she-turns-100-1508289

Fuhr, Lizzy. (2015, January 9) *We Can't Get Enough of These Fit and Fabulous Senior Citizens.* Pop Sugar Fitness. https://www.popsugar.com/fitness/inspiring-fit-seniors-36215726

Sanders, Corinne. (2019, July 19) *12 Incredible Senior Athletes Who are Proving that Age is Just a Number.* Inspire More. https://www.inspiremore.com/inspiring-senior-athletes-humana/

Loar, J. (2011). *Goddesses for Every Day: Exploring the Wisdom and Power of the Divine Feminine Around the World.* New World Library.

Made in United States
Cleveland, OH
26 May 2025